CHRONIC MULTISYMPTOM ILLNESS IN GULF WAR VETERANS

CASE DEFINITIONS REEXAMINED

Committee on the Development of a Consensus Case Definition for Chronic Multisymptom Illness in 1990–1991 Gulf War Veterans

Board on the Health of Select Populations

INSTITUTE OF MEDICINE
OF THE NATIONAL ACADEMIES

THE NATIONAL ACADEMIES PRESS
Washington, D.C.
www.nap.edu

THE NATIONAL ACADEMIES PRESS 500 Fifth Street, NW Washington, DC 20001

NOTICE: The project that is the subject of this report was approved by the Governing Board of the National Research Council, whose members are drawn from the councils of the National Academy of Sciences, the National Academy of Engineering, and the Institute of Medicine. The members of the committee responsible for the report were chosen for their special competencies and with regard for appropriate balance.

This study was supported by Contract VA240-13-D-0024 between the National Academy of Sciences and the Department of Veterans Affairs. Any opinions, findings, conclusions, or recommendations expressed in this publication are those of the authors and do not necessarily reflect the view of the organizations or agencies that provided support for this project.

International Standard Book Number-13: 978-0-309-29876-6
International Standard Book Number-10: 0-309-29876-8

Additional copies of this report are available from the National Academies Press, 500 Fifth Street, NW, Keck 360, Washington, DC 20001; (800) 624-6242 or (202) 334-3313; http://www.nap.edu.

For more information about the Institute of Medicine, visit the IOM home page at: **www.iom.edu.**

Printed in the United States of America

The serpent has been a symbol of long life, healing, and knowledge among almost all cultures and religions since the beginning of recorded history. The serpent adopted as a logotype by the Institute of Medicine is a relief carving from ancient Greece, now held by the Staatliche Museen in Berlin.

IOM (Institute of Medicine). 2014. *Chronic Multisymptom Illness in Gulf War Veterans: Case Definitions Reexamined*. Washington, DC: The National Academies Press.

"Knowing is not enough; we must apply.
Willing is not enough; we must do."
—Goethe

INSTITUTE OF MEDICINE
OF THE NATIONAL ACADEMIES

Advising the Nation. Improving Health.

THE NATIONAL ACADEMIES

Advisers to the Nation on Science, Engineering, and Medicine

The **National Academy of Sciences** is a private, nonprofit, self-perpetuating society of distinguished scholars engaged in scientific and engineering research, dedicated to the furtherance of science and technology and to their use for the general welfare. Upon the authority of the charter granted to it by the Congress in 1863, the Academy has a mandate that requires it to advise the federal government on scientific and technical matters. Dr. Ralph J. Cicerone is president of the National Academy of Sciences.

The **National Academy of Engineering** was established in 1964, under the charter of the National Academy of Sciences, as a parallel organization of outstanding engineers. It is autonomous in its administration and in the selection of its members, sharing with the National Academy of Sciences the responsibility for advising the federal government. The National Academy of Engineering also sponsors engineering programs aimed at meeting national needs, encourages education and research, and recognizes the superior achievements of engineers. Dr. C. D. Mote, Jr., is president of the National Academy of Engineering.

The **Institute of Medicine** was established in 1970 by the National Academy of Sciences to secure the services of eminent members of appropriate professions in the examination of policy matters pertaining to the health of the public. The Institute acts under the responsibility given to the National Academy of Sciences by its congressional charter to be an adviser to the federal government and, upon its own initiative, to identify issues of medical care, research, and education. Dr. Harvey V. Fineberg is president of the Institute of Medicine.

The **National Research Council** was organized by the National Academy of Sciences in 1916 to associate the broad community of science and technology with the Academy's purposes of furthering knowledge and advising the federal government. Functioning in accordance with general policies determined by the Academy, the Council has become the principal operating agency of both the National Academy of Sciences and the National Academy of Engineering in providing services to the government, the public, and the scientific and engineering communities. The Council is administered jointly by both Academies and the Institute of Medicine. Dr. Ralph J. Cicerone and Dr. C. D. Mote, Jr., are chair and vice chair, respectively, of the National Research Council.

www.national-academies.org

COMMITTEE ON THE DEVELOPMENT OF A CONSENSUS CASE DEFINITION FOR CHRONIC MULTISYMPTOM ILLNESS IN 1990–1991 GULF WAR VETERANS

KENNETH SHINE (*Chair*), Special Adviser to the Chancellor, University of Texas System, Austin, TX

FLOYD E. BLOOM, Professor Emeritus, Molecular and Integrative Neuroscience Department, The Scripps Research Institute, La Jolla, CA

KARON FRANCES COOK, Research Associate Professor, Northwestern University Feinberg School of Medicine, Chicago, IL

DEBORAH A. CORY-SLECHTA, Professor, Department of Environmental Medicine, School of Medicine and Dentistry, University of Rochester, NY

FRED FRIEDBERG, Research Associate Professor, Department of Psychiatry and Behavioral Science, Stony Brook University, Stony Brook, NY

JOANNA G. KATZMAN, Director, University of New Mexico Pain Center and Associate Professor, Department of Neurosurgery, University of New Mexico School of Medicine, Albuquerque, NM

HOWARD M. KIPEN, Professor of Environmental and Occupational Medicine and Chief, Clinical Research and Occupational Medicine Division, Rutgers-Robert Wood Johnson Medical School, Piscataway, NJ

JEANNIE-MARIE S. LEOUTSAKOS, Assistant Professor, Director, Psychiatry Biostatistics and Methodology Core, Johns Hopkins University School of Medicine, Baltimore, MD

JAMES L. LEVENSON, Professor of Psychiatry, Internal Medicine and Surgery, Virginia Commonwealth University, Richmond, VA

CATHERINE LOMEN-HOERTH, Director, ALS Center, Professor of Neurology, University of California, San Francisco, Medical Center, San Francisco, CA

THOMAS J. MASON, Professor, Department of Environmental and Occupational Health, College of Public Health, Department of Internal Medicine, College of Medicine, University of South Florida, Tampa, FL

LINDA ANH B. NGUYEN, Clinical Assistant Professor, Director, GI Motility and Neurogastroenterology, Stanford University, Palo Alto, CA

F. JAVIER NIETO, Helfaer Professor of Public Health, Professor of Population Health Sciences and Family Medicine, University of Wisconsin, School of Medicine and Public Health, Madison, WI

ANNE LOUISE OAKLANDER, Associate Professor of Neurology, Harvard Medical School, Assistant in Pathology (Neuropathology), Massachusetts General Hospital, Boston, MA

RON F. TEICHMAN, Teichman Occupational Health Associates, Inc., West Orange, NJ

SUZANNE D. VERNON, Scientific Director, The CFIDS Association of America, Charlotte, NC

IOM Staff

CAROLYN FULCO, Scholar
RENEE WLORDCZYK, Associate Program Officer (*until August 2013*)
CARY HAVER, Associate Program Officer
NORMAN GROSSBLATT, Senior Editor
JOSEPH GOODMAN, Senior Program Assistant
SULVIA DOJA, Senior Program Assistant
DORIS ROMERO, Financial Associate
FREDERICK ERDTMANN, Director, Board on the Health of Select Populations

Consultants

MIRIAM DAVIS, Independent Consultant, Silver Spring, MD
ANDREW KAYSER, Ernest Gallo Clinic & Research Center, University of California, San Francisco

REVIEWERS

This report has been reviewed in draft form by persons chosen for their diverse perspectives and technical expertise in accordance with procedures approved by the National Research Council's Report Review Committee. The purpose of this independent review is to provide candid and critical comments that will assist the institution in making its published report as sound as possible and to ensure that the report meets institutional standards of objectivity, evidence, and responsiveness to the study charge. The review comments and draft manuscript remain confidential to protect the integrity of the deliberative process. We thank the following for their review of this report:

John C. Bailar, University of Chicago
Dan G. Blazer, Duke University Medical Center
Kenneth W. Kizer, University of California, Davis
David Korn, Harvard University
Kurt Kroenke, Indiana University School of Medicine
Eric B. Larson, Group Health Research Institute
Stephen R. Mitchell, Georgetown University School of Medicine
Rebecca Nugent, Carnegie Mellon University
Tyler Smith, National University
Simon Wessely, Kings College London

Although the reviewers listed above have provided many constructive comments and suggestions, they were not asked to endorse the conclusions or recommendations, nor did they see the final draft of the report before its release. The review of the report was overseen by **Huda Akil,** University of Michigan, and **Harold C. Sox,** Dartmouth Institute for Health Policy and Clinical Practice. Appointed by the National Research Council and the Institute of Medicine, they were responsible for making certain that an independent examination of the report was carried out in accordance with institutional procedures and that all review comments were carefully considered. Responsibility for the final content of the report rests entirely with the authoring committee and the institution.

CONTENTS

SUMMARY

More than 2 decades have passed since the 1990–1991 conflict in the Persian Gulf. During the intervening years, some Gulf War veterans have experienced various unexplained symptoms that many associate with service in the gulf region, but no specific exposure has been definitively associated with symptoms. Numerous researchers have described the pattern of signs and symptoms found in deployed Gulf War veterans and noted that they report unexplained symptoms at higher rates than nondeployed veterans or veterans deployed elsewhere during the same period. Gulf War veterans have consistently shown a higher level of morbidity than the nondeployed, in some cases with severe and debilitating consequences. However, efforts to define a unique illness or syndrome in Gulf War veterans have failed, as have attempts to develop a uniformly accepted case definition.

BACKGROUND

On August 2, 1990, Iraqi armed forces invaded Kuwait; within 5 days, the United States had begun to deploy troops to Southwest Asia in Operation Desert Shield. Intense air attacks against the Iraqi armed forces began on January 16, 1991, and opened a phase of the conflict known as Operation Desert Storm. Those two operations, although brief, exposed US and coalition forces to an array of biologic and chemical agents; for example, oil-well fires became visible in satellite images as early as February 9, 1991. The ground war began on February 23; by February 28, the war was over; an official cease-fire was signed in April 1991. The oil-well fires were extinguished by November 1991. The last troops to participate in the ground war returned home on June 13, 1991. In all, about 697,000 US troops had been deployed to the Persian Gulf area during the two operations.[1] Although the military operations were considered successful, with few battle injuries and deaths, veterans soon began reporting numerous health problems that they attributed to their participation in the Gulf War. Most of the men and women who served in the Gulf War returned to normal activities without serious health problems, but many experienced an array of unexplained symptoms, such as fatigue, muscle and joint pain, loss of concentration, forgetfulness, headache, respiratory complaints, rashes, sleep disturbances, and gastrointestinal distress.

[1]Henceforth, the two operations—Desert Storm and Desert Shield—will be referred to as the Gulf War.

Charge to the Committee

The Department of Veterans Affairs (VA) provided the charge to the committee:

An ad hoc committee will develop a case definition for chronic multisymptom illness (CMI)[2] as it pertains to the 1990–1991 Gulf War Veteran population. The committee will comprehensively review, evaluate, and summarize the available scientific and medical literature regarding symptoms for CMI among the 1991 Gulf War Veterans.

In addition to reviewing and summarizing the available scientific and medical literature regarding symptoms and case definitions for CMI among Gulf War Veterans, the committee will evaluate the terminology currently used in referring to CMI in Gulf War Veterans and recommend appropriate usage.

How the Committee Approached Its Charge

The IOM appointed a committee of 16 experts to carry out the task. The committee members have expertise in occupational medicine, biostatistics, psychometrics, epidemiology, basic science, clinical medicine, toxicology, psychiatry, neurology, gastroenterology, and sociology. Some of the committee members treated Gulf War veterans when they came to their clinics or practices, and one committee members' practice is devoted solely to Gulf War and other veterans. The committee also consulted with an expert in brain imaging because that field was not represented on the committee.

The committee members directed the staff to conduct an extensive search of the extant peer-reviewed literature. PubMed was searched for all references related to the 1990–1991 Gulf War. Initially, more than 5,000 papers were retrieved; after elimination of duplicates, 2,033 unique papers remained. The titles and abstracts of those papers were reviewed, and 718 were selected for more rigorous review. The committee members divided the work by reading papers related to their expertise. The papers that were reviewed included all health outcomes that have been noted in Gulf War veterans, for example, mortality, hospitalization, neurologic symptoms, respiratory symptoms, gastrointestinal symptoms, pain, birth defects and fertility, cancer, mental-health conditions, and overlapping syndromes. In an effort to characterize the symptomatology associated with CMI, the focus of the committee's review is on studies of symptoms not associated with diagnosed medical or psychiatric conditions; the focus is on studies of symptom-reporting in Gulf War veterans. The committee agreed early on that a determination of the etiology of CMI was outside the scope of its charge. Thus, the committee did not consider toxicologic or exposure studies.

The committee held one open meeting, in which members heard from veterans, government officials, researchers, clinicians who treat Gulf War veterans, and members of the VA Research Advisory Committee. The meeting increased the committee's awareness of the variety of symptoms being experienced by the Gulf War veterans. In addition, the vigorous discussions with the veterans and researchers were invaluable for increasing the committee members' understanding of the complexity of issues involved in its task.

---

[2]The committee uses the term chronic multisymptom illness throughout the report, as defined in the statement of work, when referring to the symptom complex in Gulf War veterans.

ADDRESSING CHRONIC MULTISYMPTOM ILLNESS IN GULF WAR VETERANS

Although many Gulf War veterans suffer from an array of health problems and symptoms (such as fatigue, muscle and joint pain, memory loss, and gastrointestinal disorders), those health issues are not necessarily specific to any identified disease and are not satisfactorily classified by standard diagnostic coding systems. Population-based studies have found a higher prevalence of symptom reporting in Gulf War veterans than in nondeployed Gulf War veterans or other control groups (Goss Gilroy Inc., 1998; Iowa Persian Gulf Study Group, 1997; Unwin et al., 1999). The wide variation in types of symptoms reported by Gulf War veterans has complicated efforts to determine whether there is a unique Gulf War syndrome or whether symptom patterns are consistent with other known symptom-based disorders. Consequently, the array of symptoms suffered by many Gulf War veterans does not often point to an obvious diagnosis, etiology, or specific treatment.

The search for a definitive cause of CMI also has been difficult. The veterans of the 1990–1991 Gulf War were exposed to an impressive array of biologic and chemical agents. Numerous studies have been conducted over the past 20 years to determine an etiology based on many possible exposures, such as exposures to pyridostigmine bromide, anthrax vaccination, tent-heater fumes, oil-fire smoke, and chemical odors (Wolfe et al., 2002); jet fuel (Bell et al., 2005); low concentrations of sarin and cyclosarin (Chao et al., 2011); and combinations of organophosphate pesticides, chemical nerve agents, DEET insect repellent, and pyridostigmine bromide (Haley et al., 1997, 1999). However, exposures during the Gulf War were not reliably measured (or necessarily measured at all), and most often exposures have been evaluated through surveys or health examinations some years after they occurred (Gray et al., 2004). The association between retrospective recall of exposures and self-reported health outcomes is subject to recall bias. No coherent mechanism of action or definitive causal relationship between the exposures and the array of symptoms reported has been established (Barrett et al., 2002).

Even the terminology used over the years has at times been perplexing. Initially, the term *Gulf War syndrome* was used, and later numerous other terms appeared in the medical and scientific literature, such as *Gulf War illness*, *unexplained illness*, *medically unexplained symptoms* or *medically unexplained physical symptoms*, and *chronic multisymptom illness*. Furthermore, many of the symptoms of CMI overlap with symptoms of other diseases and ill-defined conditions, such as fibromyalgia (FM) and chronic fatigue syndrome (CFS). As noted by Ismail and Lewis (2006), when several symptoms are reported together in the absence of evidence of a physical cause, they are often termed medically unexplained syndromes. To add to the difficulty in defining CMI and finding a common etiology, the literature contains a number of discussions that refer to different postwar syndromes as possible explanations for the illnesses in Gulf War veterans (e.g., Engel, 2004; Hyams et al., 1996).

Many similarities between previously identified postwar syndromes and CMI were noted. More generally, all modern wars have been associated with medically unexplained symptoms or syndromes (Jones et al., 2002). After military personnel are deployed to war zones, some of them will have such illnesses when they return. A systematic comparison of UK pension files from previous wars (the Boer War, World War I, and World War II) with clinical files from the Gulf War found that CMI is similar to many postconflict syndromes. During the Boer War, soldiers complained primarily of fatigue, rheumatic pains, weakness, shortness of breath, rapid heart rate, headache, and dizziness. In World War I and World War II, primary symptom complaints were chest pain, breathlessness, dizziness, fatigue, and to a lesser extent headache and anxiety (King's College London, 2010).

Case Definitions of Chronic Multisymptom Illness in Gulf War Veterans

One of the tasks of the committee was to examine the peer-reviewed literature specific to deployed Gulf War veterans' symptomatology in an effort to develop or identify a case definition that will show adequate sensitivity and specificity for research and treatment purposes. In the numerous symptom studies reviewed by the committee, the array of symptoms reported makes it difficult to identify hallmark characteristics of the illness. In addition, the symptoms detailed in Gulf War veterans are shared by other symptom-based disorders such as CFS and FM and are seen in the general adult population. There are no objective diagnostic criteria (such as laboratory abnormalities or characteristic physical signs), so diagnosing symptom-based conditions, such as CMI, often must depend on the exclusion of other causes. Thus, specificity becomes a major limitation in developing a case definition of CMI. As noted by Hyams (1998), specificity requires a low proportion of false positives; however, without diagnostic criteria that exclude well-recognized medical and psychiatric causes of symptoms and distinguish them from other symptom-based conditions, a specific diagnosis has not been possible.

The committee recognizes the difficulty of establishing a consensus case definition of CMI, given the lack of uniform symptoms, the variety of symptoms, and the long onset and duration. However, CMI is an important cause of disability in Gulf War veterans and the lack of a consensus case definition poses problems for those who are suffering with this illness. The absence of a consensus case definition is a fundamental weakness of CMI research in that the lack of an agreed on case definition can make it difficult to identify cases and controls. It prevents the accurate estimation of the burden of illness in the veteran population, the use of generalizable results, the accumulation of valid information about the condition, and the effectiveness of treatment.

In a clinical setting, the absence of an agreed upon case definition of CMI not only can result in considerable uncertainty about the diagnosis, but might limit the ability to select and administer effective treatments. Practically, that means that there will be some veterans misdiagnosed either as having or not having CMI and the course of treatments might not be helpful. That can have an adverse effect on the health of the veteran with respect to worrying about the lack of improvement, possible side effects of treatment, and the cost of treatment. The impact on health care services may also be considerable, and whether such treatments constitute an effective use of limited resources should be a cause of concern.

For those reasons, the committee believes that supporting the development of a case definition or the adoption of a current definition will move the field forward. The committee also recognizes that as the knowledge base changes over time, a case definition will need to evolve as has occurred in other symptom-based conditions, such as irritable bowel syndrome, CFS, and FM.

GULF WAR SYMPTOM STUDIES

Researchers began to assemble cohorts of Gulf War veterans in the first few years after the war; others were assembled later. Most of the studies compare sizable groups of deployed veterans with groups of veterans who were not deployed during the same period as the Gulf War (often referred to as era veterans) or who were deployed to locations other than the Persian Gulf, such as Bosnia (referred to as deployed elsewhere). In addition, a number of volunteer registries were assembled by the US Department of Defense and Department of Veterans Affairs and by governments whose forces were included in the Gulf War coalition to study their veterans' health.

The committee focused on those symptom studies, rather than on studies of well-characterized diagnosed medical and psychiatric conditions, and they provide the foundation for the committee's understanding of the symptomatology in the Gulf War veterans. A review of all the studies indicates that many Gulf War veterans suffer from an array of health problems and symptoms (for example, fatigue, muscle and joint pain, memory loss, gastrointestinal disorders, and rashes) that are not specific to any disease and are not easily classified with standard diagnostic coding systems. In studies since the mid-1990s, researchers have found a higher prevalence of self-reported and clinically verified symptoms in Gulf War veterans than in nondeployed Gulf War–era veterans or other control groups. Veterans of the Gulf War from Australia, Canada, Danish, the United Kingdom, and the United States report higher rates and increased severity of nearly all symptoms or sets of symptoms than their nondeployed counterparts; that finding was reported consistently in every study that the committee reviewed. However, Gulf War veterans do not all experience the same array of symptoms, and the symptoms reported are also found in the nondeployed.

General Limitations of Gulf War Studies

The cohort studies of Gulf War veterans have contributed greatly to the understanding of veterans' health, but limitations are commonly encountered in observational epidemiologic studies. They include selection biases that limit the studies' control for potential confounding factors, self-reporting of health outcomes and exposures affected by recall bias, outcome misclassification, and reporting bias.[3]

Other limitations of the body of evidence are that studies might be too narrow in their assessment of health status, the measurement instruments might have been too insensitive to detect abnormalities that affect deployed veterans, and the period of investigation might have been too brief to detect health outcomes that have a long latency or require many years to progress to the point where disability, hospitalization, or death occurs.

Finally, research into the health effects of Gulf War deployment is limited by the interval between the war and the conduct of studies. Many studies were conducted years after the war, and this limits the ability to determine when symptoms developed and to detect causal associations; for example, some of the earliest assessments were conducted in 1993 by Pierce (1997) and Wolfe et al. (1998), in 1994 by Gray et al. (1999), and in 1995 by Fukuda et al. (1998). The delay also allows dissemination of speculation by the news media and others that may affect veterans' recall (Hotopf and Wessely, 2005).

[3]Biases previously described by the IOM (2006, 2010).

THE USE OF FACTOR ANALYSIS IN STUDIES OF CHRONIC MULTISYMPTOM ILLNESS

In an effort to understand the symptomatology in Gulf War veterans, researchers began to use statistical analyses (specifically, factor and cluster analyses) to evaluate whether symptoms found in Gulf War veterans might constitute a unique syndrome. Factor analysis is a statistical method for conducting structural analyses of datasets. The data used in factor-analytic studies can be people's responses to a set of items or list of symptoms with respect to their presence or absence and their severity. Factor analysis also was used to inform a case definition. In attempting to reduce the amount of data that were gathered (the large and varied number of symptoms), researchers used factor analysis so that a structure that included substantially fewer factors than symptoms could be proposed.

Factor Analysis for Case Definition

Factor-analytic studies have facilitated and clarified comparisons of symptom prevalence and severity between deployed and nondeployed, but they have been less useful in specifying a case definition of CMI. The results of factor analyses do not differentiate among groups of people and cannot create a case definition. That fact has been obscured because investigators often operationalize a case definition by dichotomizing factor scores obtained from a factor-analytic model. However, people do not have factors; everyone will have a score on each factor, but dichotomization of factor scores to define a "case" is a postprocessing decision made by the investigator and is not a direct result of the factor-analytic model.

The studies that have used factor analysis to investigate symptoms in Gulf War veterans have used several strategies. Some studies used statistical testing of the hypothesis that the factor structures of deployed and nondeployed veteran populations are significantly different (that is, testing the null hypothesis that the structures are the same) (Ismail et al., 1999). Others relied exclusively on descriptive statistical techniques, such as correlations among factors, factor scores, or factor loadings (Doebbeling et al., 2000; Haley et al., 1997; Kang et al., 2002). Finally, a number of studies used "visual inspection" to discern differences between the factor structures for deployed and nondeployed groups (Knoke et al., 2000; Nisenbaum et al., 2004; Shapiro et al., 2002).

Factor analysis and cluster analysis may be useful for making sense of the large number of symptoms potentially associated with CMI. However, the findings that result from using those methods must be validated against other observed variables. The choice of variables to include in the factor-analytic model is critical, and omission of key symptoms will result in models that do not capture the most salient features of CMI. In addition, the validity of factor analysis or cluster analysis depends on the quality of data. Methodologic flaws in such studies can bias results (Ismail and Lewis, 2006). The committee notes that neither factor analysis nor cluster analysis alone can directly produce a case definition.

DISCUSSION OF EXISTING CASE DEFINITIONS

The case definition studies do not all consistently identify key elements of a case definition, which might include, for example, period of onset, duration, frequency, severity, exposure, exclusionary criteria, or a uniform set of symptoms. There are no clinically validated tests or measures for diagnosing CMI. And the symptoms of CMI are not unique to Gulf War–

deployed veterans, although they occur in the deployed at a higher frequency and severity than in nondeployed era veterans or those deployed elsewhere. That is evidenced by higher prevalences of a variety of symptoms, as noted in the cohort studies. Thus, the committee has concluded that the available evidence is insufficient to develop a new case definition of CMI.

To move the field forward, however, the committee developed an approach based on its evaluation of the CMI literature and its collective judgment. In its review of CMI symptomatology, factor analyses, and case definitions, the committee noted similarities throughout the body of literature. A common set of symptoms has been identified in the case-definition studies (albeit not necessarily using the same terminology) that includes symptoms of fatigue, pain, and neurocognitive dysfunction (see Table S.1).

TABLE S.1 Case Definitions of Chronic Multisymptom Illness Used in Gulf War Veteran Studies

Definition	Symptoms—must have signs, symptoms, or complaints that fit at least	Duration	Onset	Exclusions	Severity
Haley—clinical (Haley et al., 1997)	5 of 8 signs or symptoms: 1) fatigue 2) arthralgia or low back pain 3) headache 4) intermittent diarrhea without bloody stools 5) neuropsychiatric complaints of forgetfulness, difficulty in concentrating, depression, memory loss, or easy irritability 6) difficulty in sleeping 7) low-grade fever 8) weight loss			Must be denied a physician's diagnosis of other medical and psychiatric illnesses that could cause the symptoms	
Haley—factor analysis (Haley et al., 1997)	Cases are defined mathematically by using factor scores calculated with weights; cases with factor scores >1.5 are identified as having a syndrome (a factor derived with the same factor analysis); cases may have multiple syndromes				
CDC (Fukuda et al., 1998)	1 or more from at least 2 of the following categories: 1) fatigue 2) mood and cognition (symptoms of feeling depressed, difficulty in remembering or concentrating, feeling moody, feeling anxious, trouble in finding words, or difficulty in sleeping) 3) musculoskeletal (symptoms of joint pain, joint stiffness, or	≥6 months			Mild, moderate, or severe by self-report

Definition	Symptoms—must have signs, symptoms, or complaints that fit at least	Duration	Onset	Exclusions	Severity
	muscle pain)				
Kansas (Steele, 2000)	3 of 6 domains: 1) fatigue and sleep problems 2) pain symptoms 3) neurologic, cognitive, or mood symptoms 4) gastrointestinal symptoms 5) respiratory symptoms 6) skin symptoms	Chronic	Since 1990	Symptom reporting must be in the absence of diagnosed exclusionary conditions; only respondents who have at least 1 moderately severe symptom or 2 or more symptoms within a group were considered to have a high level of symptoms in the group	Mild, moderate, or severe by self-report
Portland (Bourdette et al., 2001; Spencer et al., 1998)	Symptoms in 1 of 3 categories: 1) fatigue (unexplained fatigue and at least 4 of the following: fevers and chills; new kinds of headache; unrefreshing sleep; tender glands in the neck, jaw, or groin; changes in memory or difficulty in concentrating; sore throat; painful joints; unexplained weakness in many muscles; persistent muscle aches; prolonged fatigue; and feeling of illness lasting longer than 1 day after mild exercise) 2) cognitive and psychologic symptoms, including memory loss, confusion, inability to concentrate, mood swings, and sleep difficulties 3) musculoskeletal symptoms, including back pain, persistent muscle aches or pains, painful joints, swollen joints, joint stiffness, and pain after exertion	≥1 month within the 3 previous months	During or after deployment to the Persian Gulf		
VA (Kang et al., 2009)	Might include things like fatigue, muscle or joint pain, headache, memory problems, digestive problems, respiratory problems, skin problems, or any other unexplained symptoms that may	≥6 months		Must not be adequately explained by conventional medical or psychiatric	

Definition	Symptoms—must have signs, symptoms, or complaints that fit at least	Duration	Onset	Exclusions	Severity
	sometimes be diagnosed as chronic fatigue syndrome, fibromyalgia, irritable bowel syndrome, or multiple chemical sensitivity			diagnoses	

NOTE: Other elements of case definitions (such as laboratory criteria and exposure) not reported.

Furthermore symptoms were regularly reported with higher frequency in Gulf War veterans than in nondeployed era veterans or veterans who were deployed elsewhere; they include gastrointestinal, respiratory, and dermatologic symptoms (those were in addition to the fatigue, pain, and neurocognitive symptoms already identified). The committee recognized that two *existing* definitions—the Centers for Disease Control and Prevention (CDC) definition and the Kansas definition (see Table S.1)—capture the array of symptoms most commonly identified. The CDC definition requires one or more symptoms in at least two of the fatigue, pain, and mood and cognition categories to identify a case. The Kansas definition requires symptoms in at least three of the domains of fatigue or sleep, pain, neurologic or cognitive or mood, gastrointestinal, respiratory, and skin to identify a case. Thus, both definitions capture the array of symptoms highlighted by the evidence. The CDC case definition, which has been widely used by researchers, identifies 29–60% of US Gulf War–deployed veterans as CMI cases depending on the population studied, whereas the Kansas definition identifies 34% in the population studied (Kansas Gulf War veterans). However, the two definitions have important differences. The CDC definition has the greatest concordance with all the other definitions (see Table S.1) but is less restrictive than the Kansas definition. The CDC definition requires fewer symptoms, does not have any exclusionary criteria, and might identify a case without physical symptoms. In contrast, the Kansas definition will define fewer veterans as cases. The committee also noted particular strengths of each definition, including the CDC definition's inclusion of severity indicators and the Kansas definition's exclusionary criteria. In the committee's judgment, however, neither definition has been sufficiently validated. Given the absence of validators, the committee recommends, with some reticence, the use of two current case definitions. The CDC and Kansas definitions are the best reflection of the symptom complexes demonstrated by the Gulf War veterans. The committee recognizes that the definitions were developed in different study populations and that they differ in their sensitivity and specificity. However, in the committee's judgment, those two definitions will provide the VA with a framework to further research and treatment.

In conclusion, the committee saw merits in both the CDC and Kansas definitions, but the weight of the evidence does not currently support the use of one rather than the other for all purposes. Given the differences, the committee notes the importance of choosing a definition that is based on specific needs. For example, the CDC definition may not be suitable for research that requires a more narrowly defined study population whereas the Kansas definition may identify too few cases and compromise statistical power. Another consideration in choosing a definition is the ability to adapt it for use in clinical settings.

RECOMMENDATIONS

Evidence is lacking in the studies reviewed to characterize most elements of a case definition (for example, onset, duration, severity, and laboratory findings) with certainty. Without that information, the committee could not develop a new definition for CMI. Furthermore, because that information is lacking, few of the studies that proposed definitions were able to describe many of the elements of a case definition. Although all the studies describe clinical features (symptoms), many of the other criteria are not discussed. Therefore, the committee cannot recommend one specific case definition over another. But it does recommend the consideration of two case definitions on the basis of their concordance with the evidence and their ability to identify specific symptoms commonly reported by Gulf War veterans.

There is a set of symptoms (fatigue, pain, neurocognitive) that are reported in all the studies that have been reviewed. The CDC definition captures those three symptoms; the Kansas definition also captures them, but it also includes the symptoms reported most frequently by Gulf War veterans. Other case-definition studies report additional symptoms that are not seen with the same frequency or in all studies. Thus, the committee identified the CDC definition (Fukuda et al., 1998) and the Kansas definition (Steele, 2000) as the two that capture the array of symptoms most frequently reported by veterans as evidenced by the studies reviewed.

The committee recommends that the Department of Veterans Affairs consider the use of the Centers for Disease Control and Prevention and Kansas definitions because they capture the most commonly reported symptoms.

Neither definition addresses all the key features of a case definition, such as symptom onset, duration, severity, frequency of symptoms, and exclusionary criteria. Identifying those features will contribute to a more accurate case definition. Those features were not regularly reported in the studies considered. It is important to acknowledge that the two definitions, although they cover the most common symptoms, do not reflect the complete array of symptoms reported by Gulf War veterans. Although a standard set of criteria regarding time (a defined period of onset), place, exposures, and clinical and laboratory findings would have been useful; given the lag in time between first reports of illness and epidemiologic study, lack of exposure monitoring, and the absence of validated laboratory tests, it is no longer possible to define many of the typical elements associated with a case definition. However, review of existing data sets might prove useful in detailing some of the needed information.

The committee recommends that the Department of Veterans Affairs, to the extent possible, systematically assess existing data to identify additional features of chronic multisymptom illness, such as onset, duration, severity, frequency of symptoms, and exclusionary criteria to produce a more robust case definition.

Finally, VA asked the committee to evaluate the terminology used in referring to CMI in 1990–1991 Gulf War veterans and to recommend appropriate terminology. Multiple terms have been used over the past 2 decades. Initially, *Gulf War syndrome* was used, but *syndrome* indicates a new group of signs and symptoms not previously seen in medicine (IOM, 2000; King's College London, 2010). The Gulf War veterans report more symptoms and with greater frequency and severity than nondeployed veterans or veterans who were deployed elsewhere, but the types and patterns of symptoms are the same in all groups, and this suggests that no unique syndrome is associated with Gulf War deployment.

Although *chronic multisymptom illness* is descriptive of the heterogeneity of the symptoms, it is not specific to the population and its unique experience. Thus, to capture the population of interest and the symptoms, a preferred term is *Gulf War illness*. Illnesses are sometimes named after the geographic area or the group in which they were first identified without meaning to convey a sole etiology (for example, the 1918 influenza pandemic referred to as the Spanish flu, the 1968 and 1969 influenza outbreaks referred to as the Hong Kong flu, and pneumonia in legionnaires referred to as Legionnaire's disease). The committee's recommendation reflects both the geographic area and the unique experiences of this group of veterans. *Gulf War illness* has been used by many researchers to identify the array of symptoms expressed by Gulf War veterans. Its consistent use in the literature might reduce confusion.

> **The committee recommends that the Department of Veterans Affairs use the term *Gulf War illness* rather than *chronic multisymptom illness*.**

REFERENCES

Barrett, D. H., G. C. Gray, B. N. Doebbeling, D. J. Clauw, and W. C. Reeves. 2002. Prevalence of symptoms and symptom-based conditions among Gulf War veterans: Current status of research findings. *Epidemiologic Reviews* 24(2):218-227.

Bell, I. R., A. J. Brooks, C. M. Baldwin, M. Fernandez, A. J. Figueredo, and M. L. Witten. 2005. JP-8 jet fuel exposure and divided attention test performance in 1991 Gulf War veterans. *Aviation Space and Environmental Medicine* 76(12):1136-1144.

Bourdette, D. N., L. A. McCauley, A. Barkhuizen, W. Johnston, M. Wynn, S. K. Joos, D. Storzbach, T. Shuell, and D. Sticker. 2001. Symptom factor analysis, clinical findings, and functional status in a population-based case control study of Gulf War unexplained illness. *Journal of Occupational and Environmental Medicine* 43(12):1026-1040.

Chao, L. L., L. Abadjian, J. Hlavin, D. J. Meyerhoff, and M. W. Weiner. 2011. Effects of low-level sarin and cyclosarin exposure and Gulf War illness on brain structure and function: A study at 4t. *Neurotoxicology* 32(6):814-822.

Doebbeling, B. N., W. R. Clarke, D. Watson, J. C. Torner, R. F. Woolson, M. D. Voelker, D. H. Barrett, and D. A. Schwartz. 2000. Is there a Persian Gulf War syndrome? Evidence from a large population-based survey of veterans and nondeployed controls. *American Journal of Medicine* 108(9):695-704.

Engel, C. C., Jr. 2004. Post-war syndromes: Illustrating the impact of the social psyche on notions of risk, responsibility, reason, and remedy. *Journal of the American Academy of Psychoanalysis and Dynamic Psychiatry* 32(2):321-334; discussion 335-343.

Fukuda, K., R. Nisenbaum, G. Stewart, W. W. Thompson, L. Robin, R. M. Washko, D. L. Noah, D. H. Barrett, B. Randall, B. L. Herwaldt, A. C. Mawle, and W. C. Reeves. 1998. Chronic multisymptom illness affecting Air Force veterans of the Gulf War. *Journal of the American Medical Association* 280(11):981-988.

Goss Gilroy Inc. 1998. *Health study of Canadian Forces Personnel Involved in the 1991 Conflict in the Persian Gulf.* Ottawa, Canada: Goss Gilroy Inc. Department of National Defence.

Gray, G. C., G. D. Gackstetter, H. K. Kang, J. T. Graham, and K. C. Scott. 2004. After more than 10 years of Gulf War veteran medical evaluations, what have we learned? *American Journal of Preventive Medicine* 26(5):443-452.

Gray, G. C., K. S. Kaiser, A. W. Hawksworth, F. W. Hall, and E. Barrett-Connor. 1999. Increased postwar symptoms and psychological morbidity among U.S. Navy Gulf War veterans. *American Journal of Tropical Medicine and Hygiene* 60(5):758-766.

Haley, R. W., T. L. Kurt, and J. Hom. 1997. Is there a Gulf War syndrome? Searching for syndromes by factor analysis of symptoms. *Journal of the American Medical Association* 277(3):215-222. [Erratum appears in *Journal of the American Medical Association* 1997; 278(5):388.]

Haley, R. W., S. Billecke, and B. N. La Du. 1999. Association of low PON1 type Q (type A) arylesterase activity with neurologic symptom complexes in Gulf War veterans. *Toxicology and Applied Pharmacology* 157(3):227-233.

Hotopf, M., and S. Wessely. 2005. Can epidemiology clear the fog of war? Lessons from the 1990–91 Gulf War. *International Journal of Epidemiology* 34(4):791-800.

Hyams, K. C. 1998. Developing case definitions for symptom-based conditions: The problem of specificity. *Epidemiologic Reviews* 20(2):148-156.

Hyams, K. C., F. S. Wignall, and R. Roswell. 1996. War syndromes and their evaluation: From the U.S. Civil War to the Persian Gulf War. *Annals of Internal Medicine* 125(5):398-405.

IOM (Institute of Medicine). 2000. *Gulf War and Health, Volume 1: Depleted Uranium, Pyrodostigmine Bromide, Sarin, Vaccines*. Washington, DC: National Academy Press.

IOM. 2006. *Gulf War and Health, Volume 4: Health Effects of Serving in the Gulf War*. Washington, DC: The National Academies Press.

IOM. 2010. *Gulf War and Health, Volume 8: Update of Health Effects of Serving in the Gulf War*. Washington, DC: The National Academies Press.

Iowa Persian Gulf Study Group. 1997. Self-reported illness and health status among Gulf War veterans: A population-based study. *Journal of the American Medical Association* 277(3):238-245.

Ismail, K., and G. Lewis. 2006. Multi-symptom illnesses, unexplained illness and Gulf War syndrome. *Philosophical Transactions of the Royal Society B: Biological Sciences* 361(1468):543-551.

Ismail, K., B. Everitt, N. Blatchley, L. Hull, C. Unwin, A. David, and S. Wessely. 1999. Is there a Gulf War syndrome? *Lancet* 353(9148):179-182.

Jones, E., R. Hodgins-Vermaas, H. McCartney, B. Everitt, C. Beech, D. Poynter, I. Palmer, K. Hyams, and S. Wessely. 2002. Post-combat syndromes from the Boer War to the Gulf War: A cluster analysis of their nature and attribution. *British Medical Journal* 324(7333):321-324.

Kang, H. K., C. M. Mahan, K. Y. Lee, F. M. Murphy, S. J. Simmens, H. A. Young, and P. H. Levine. 2002. Evidence for a deployment-related Gulf War syndrome by factor analysis. *Archives of Environmental Health* 57(1):61-68.

Kang, H. K., B. Li, C. M. Mahan, S. A. Eisen, and C. C. Engel. 2009. Health of US veterans of 1991 Gulf War: A follow-up survey in 10 years. *Journal of Occupational and Environmental Medicine* 51(4):401-410.

King's College London. 2010. *King's Centre for Military Health Research: A Fifteen Year Report. What Has Been Achieved by Fifteen Years of Research into the Health of the UK Armed Forces?* University of London.

Knoke, J. D., T. C. Smith, G. C. Gray, K. S. Kaiser, and A. W. Hawksworth. 2000. Factor analysis of self-reported symptoms: Does it identify a Gulf War syndrome? *American Journal of Epidemiology* 152(4):379-388.

Nisenbaum, R., K. Ismail, S. Wessely, C. Unwin, L. Hull, and W. C. Reeves. 2004. Dichotomous factor analysis of symptoms reported by UK and US veterans of the 1991 Gulf War. *Population Health Metrics* 2.

Pierce, P. F. 1997. Physical and emotional health of Gulf War veteran women. *Aviation Space and Environmental Medicine* 68(4):317-321.

Shapiro, S. E., M. R. Lasarev, and L. McCauley. 2002. Factor analysis of Gulf War illness: What does it add to our understanding of possible health effects of deployment? *American Journal of Epidemiology* 156(6):578-585.

Spencer, P. S., L. A. McCauley, S. K. Joos, M. R. Lasarev, T. Schuell, D. Bourdette, A. Barkhuizen, W. Johnston, D. Storzbach, M. Wynn, and R. Grewenow. 1998. U.S. Gulf War veterans: Service periods in theater, differential exposures, and persistent unexplained illness. Portland Environmental Hazards Research Centre. *Toxicology Letters* 102-103:515-521.

Steele, L. 2000. Prevalence and patterns of Gulf War illness in Kansas veterans: Association of symptoms with characteristics of person, place, and time of military service. *American Journal of Epidemiology* 152(10):992-1002.

Unwin, C., N. Blatchley, W. Coker, S. Ferry, M. Hotopf, L. Hull, K. Ismail, I. Palmer, A. David, and S. Wessely. 1999. Health of UK servicemen who served in Persian Gulf War. *Lancet* 353(9148):169-178.

Wolfe, J., S. P. Proctor, J. D. Davis, M. S. Borgos, and M. J. Friedman. 1998. Health symptoms reported by Persian Gulf War veterans two years after return. *American Journal of Industrial Medicine* 33(2):104-113.

Wolfe, J., S. P. Proctor, D. J. Erickson, and H. Hu. 2002. Risk factors for multisymptom illness in US Army veterans of the Gulf War. *Journal of Occupational and Environmental Medicine* 44(3):271-281.

1

INTRODUCTION

More than 2 decades have passed since the 1990–1991 conflict in the Persian Gulf. During the intervening years, some Gulf War veterans have experienced various unexplained symptoms that many associate with service in the gulf region, but no specific exposure has been definitively associated with symptoms. Research has been hampered by a lack of exposure measurements and a lack of objective measures of health outcomes in the veterans.

Numerous researchers have described the pattern of signs and symptoms found in Gulf War veterans and noted that veterans deployed to the gulf report unexplained symptoms at higher rates than nondeployed veterans or veterans deployed elsewhere during the same period. Gulf War veterans have consistently shown a higher level of morbidity than the nondeployed, in some cases with severe and debilitating consequences.

BACKGROUND

On August 2, 1990, Iraqi armed forces invaded Kuwait; within 5 days, the United States had begun to deploy troops to Southwest Asia in Operation Desert Shield. Intense air attacks against the Iraqi armed forces began on January 16, 1991, and opened a phase of the conflict known as Operation Desert Storm. Those two operations, although brief, exposed US and coalition forces to an array of biologic and chemical agents; for example, oil-well fires became visible in satellite images as early as February 9, 1991. The ground war began on February 23; by February 28, 1991, the war was over; and an official cease-fire was signed in April 1991. The oil-well fires were extinguished by November 1991. The last troops to participate in the ground war returned home on June 13, 1991. In all, about 697,000 US troops had been deployed to the Persian Gulf area during the two operations.[1]

Although the military operations were considered successful, with few battle injuries and deaths, veterans soon began reporting numerous health problems that they attributed to their participation in the Gulf War. Most of the men and women who served in the Gulf War returned to normal activities without serious health problems, but many experienced an array of unexplained symptoms, such as fatigue, muscle and joint pain, loss of concentration, forgetfulness, headache, respiratory complaints, rashes, sleep disturbances, and gastrointestinal distress.

[1]Henceforth, the two operations—Desert Storm and Desert Shield—will be referred to as the Gulf War.

The men and women who served in the Persian Gulf region potentially were exposed to a wide variety of environmental, biologic, and chemical agents—including sand, smoke from oil-well fires, paints, solvents, insecticides, petroleum fuels and their combustion products, organophosphate nerve agents, pyridostigmine bromide (PB), depleted uranium (DU), anthrax and botulinum toxoid vaccines, and infectious diseases—in addition to psychologic and physiologic stress. In the more than 20 years that have passed since the Gulf War, veterans of that war have suffered numerous health consequences that might be related to exposure to those agents, conditions, and circumstances, although none of them has been causally linked to the Gulf War veterans' symptoms. Numerous studies and reports have investigated possible causes of Gulf War veterans' symptoms (e.g., the Institute of Medicine's Gulf War and Health series, Volumes 1 [2000], 2 [2003], and 3 [2005]; Brown, 2006; King's College, 2010).

In response to concerns about Gulf War veterans' ill health, two laws were passed: the Persian Gulf War Veterans Act of 1998 (Public Law 105-277) and the Veterans Programs Enhancement Act of 1998 (Public Law 105-368). Each law mandated studies by the National Academy of Sciences' Institute of Medicine (IOM) to examine the biologic and chemical hazards experienced in the gulf that might have been associated with the illnesses of Gulf War veterans. In the intervening years, the IOM, research organizations, and independent researchers have studied the many exposures in the gulf region and their potential for causing the array of symptoms reported by Gulf War veterans.

THE GULF WAR SETTING[2]

The pace of the buildup for the war was unprecedented. In the first 3 months, the rapid deployment of US forces by sea and air exceeded that of any previous initial US period of war. Within 5 days of the Iraqi invasion of Kuwait, the United States and other coalition countries had begun to move troops into the region. By September 15, 1990, within 6 weeks of the invasion of Kuwait, deployed American service members numbered 150,000, including nearly 50,000 reservists. Within the next month, another 60,000 troops arrived in Southwest Asia; in November, an additional 135,000 reservists and National Guard members were called up (DOD, 1992).

The Gulf War differed from previous wars in the demographic composition of military personnel and the uncertain conditions for many reservists. Of the total number deployed, almost 7% were women and about 17% were from National Guard and reserve units. Military personnel were, overall, older than those who had participated in previous wars, with a mean age of 27 years, as of 1991 (Joseph et al., 1997). Rapid mobilization exerted substantial pressures on those who were deployed, disrupting lives, separating families, and, for reserve and National Guard units, creating uncertainty about whether jobs would be available when they returned to civilian life.

[2]Adapted from *Gulf War and Health, Volume 1: Depleted Uranium, Pyridostigmine Bromide, Sarin, Vaccines* (IOM, 2000); *Gulf War and Health, Volume 2: Insecticides and Solvents* (IOM, 2003); *Gulf War and Health, Volume 3: Fuels, Combustion Products, and Propellants* (IOM, 2005).

Living Conditions

Combat troops were crowded together in warehouses and tents on arrival and then often moved to isolated desert locations with limited protection from the environmental elements. Most troops lived in tents and slept on cots lined up side by side, which afforded virtually no privacy or quiet. Sanitation was often primitive, with strains on latrines and communal washing facilities. Hot showers were infrequent, the interval between launderings of uniforms was sometimes long, and desert flies, scorpions, and snakes were a constant nuisance. Military personnel worked long hours and had few outlets for relaxation. Troops were ordered not to fraternize with local people, and alcohol was prohibited in deference to religious beliefs in the host countries. A mild, traveler's type of diarrhea affected more than 50% of the troops in some units. Fresh fruits and vegetables from neighboring countries were identified as the risk factor and were removed from the diet. Thereafter, the diet consisted mostly of packaged foods and bottled water.

For the first 2 months of troop deployment (August and September), temperatures were extremely high, as high as 115°F, with sand temperatures upwards of 150°F. Except for coastal regions, the relative humidity was less than 40%. Troops had to drink large quantities of water to prevent dehydration. Although the summer months were hot and dry, temperatures in winter (December through March) were low; wind-chill temperatures at night dropped to well below freezing. Wind and blowing sand made protection of skin and eyes imperative. Troops were not allowed to wear contact lenses except in air-conditioned areas that were protected from sand.

Environmental and Chemical Exposures

The most visually dramatic environmental event of the Gulf War was the smoke from more than 750 oil-well fires. Smoke rose and formed giant plumes that could be seen for hundreds of kilometers. There were other potential sources of exposure to petroleum-based products. Kerosene, diesel, and leaded gasoline were used in unvented tent heaters, cooking stoves, and portable generators. Petroleum products, including diesel fuels, were used to suppress sand and dust, and petroleum fuels were used for burning waste and trash.

Pesticides, including dog flea collars, were widely used by troops in the gulf to combat the region's ubiquitous insect and rodent populations. Permethrin was provided in spray cans for treating uniforms, and DEET in liquid or stick form was used as a personal mosquito and fly repellent. Other pesticides used by military personnel included methyl carbamates, organophosphates, and chlorinated hydrocarbons. Insecticides were used to control insects that are vectors of infectious diseases, such as leishmaniasis, sand fly fever, and malaria.

Many possible exposures were related to particular occupational activities in the Gulf War. Most of the occupational chemical exposures appear to have been related to repair and maintenance activities, including battery repair (corrosive liquids), cleaning or degreasing (solvents, such as chlorinated hydrocarbons), sandblasting (abrasive particles), vehicle repair (asbestos, carbon monoxide, and organic solvents), weapon repair (lead particles), and welding or cutting (chromates, nitrogen dioxide, and heated metal fumes). Troops painted vehicles and equipment used in the gulf with chemical-agent–resistant coatings either before they were shipped to the gulf or in ports in Saudi Arabia. Working conditions in the field were not ideal, and recommended occupational-hygiene standards might not have been followed at all times.

Exposure of US personnel to DU occurred as the result of friendly-fire incidents, cleanup operations, and accidents (including fires). Others may have inhaled DU dust through contact with DU-contaminated tanks or munitions. DU is 67% denser than lead, has a high melting point, is highly pyrophoric, has a tensile strength comparable with that of most steels, and is chemically highly reactive. Because of those characteristics, the US military used a layer of DU for protection in heavy-armor tanks and in weapons.

Threat of Chemical and Biologic Warfare

When US troops first arrived in the gulf, they had no way of knowing whether they would be exposed to biologic and chemical weapons. Iraq had used such weapons in fighting Iran and in attacks on the Kurdish minority in Iraq. Military leaders feared that the use of such weapons in the gulf could result in the deaths of tens of thousands of Americans. Therefore, in addition to the standard vaccinations given before military deployment, about 150,000 troops received anthrax vaccine and about 8,000 received botulinum toxoid vaccine. Troops were also given blister packs of 21 tablets of PB to protect against possible chemical warfare; they were to take PB on the orders of a commanding officer when chemical-warfare attack was believed to be imminent.

Chemical sensors and alarms were distributed throughout the region to warn of such attacks. The alarms were extremely sensitive and could be triggered by many substances, including some organic solvents, vehicle exhaust fumes, and insecticides. Although followup analysis by the Department of Defense (DOD) found no evidence of the use of chemical-warfare agents, the alarms sounded often; troops responded by donning confining protective gear and ingesting PB as an antidote to the effects of nerve gas. In addition to the alarms, there were widespread reports of dead sheep, goats, and camels, and troops were taught that those could indicate the use of chemical or biologic weapons. The sounding of the alarms, the reports of dead animals, and rumors that other units had been hit by chemical-warfare agents caused the troops to be concerned that they would be or had been exposed to the agents.

After the war, there was the potential for exposure to additional chemicals, such as sarin and cyclosarin. Unbeknownst to the troops at the time, US demolition of munitions stored in a complex in Khamisiyah, Iraq, liberated stores of sarin and cyclosarin. DOD conducted dispersion modeling to estimate exposure, but none of the models found any troops to have been exposed to concentrations above "first-noticeable-effects levels," that is, concentrations that would have been high enough to set off chemical alarms or to produce visible symptoms of acute cholinergic syndrome[3] among troops. No medical reports by the US Army Medical Corps at the time of the release were consistent with signs and symptoms of an acute exposure to sarin or cyclosarin. That is consistent with the absence of reports of symptoms of acute cholinergic syndrome by medical personnel or veterans. However, as noted in a 2004 General Accounting Office report (GAO, 2004), epidemiologic studies that use the DOD models incorporate substantial exposure misclassification because of errors in estimation of troop locations combined with uncertainty regarding plume locations. Low-level exposure could have occurred without producing acute cholinergic syndrome.

---

[3]Acute cholinergic syndrome is evident seconds to hours after exposure and usually resolves in days to months. Symptoms may include copious respiratory and oral secretions, diarrhea, vomiting, sweating, altered mental status, autonomic instability, and generalized weakness that can progress to paralysis and respiratory arrest.

CHARGE TO THE COMMITTEE

The Department of Veterans Affairs (VA) provided the charge to the committee, which is presented below:

An ad hoc committee will develop a case definition for chronic multisymptom illness (CMI)[4] as it pertains to the 1990–1991 Gulf War Veteran population. The committee will comprehensively review, evaluate, and summarize the available scientific and medical literature regarding symptoms for CMI among the 1991 Gulf War Veterans. The committee will look broadly for relevant information, including, but not limited to:

- Published peer-reviewed literature describing the symptomatology for CMI;
- Published peer-reviewed literature concerning existing case definitions for CMI among the 1990–1991 Gulf War Veteran population;
- Published peer-reviewed literature concerning existing case definitions of CMI among similar populations such as Allied military personnel; and
- Published peer-reviewed literature concerning case definitions for other populations with a similar constellation of symptoms.
- Discussions with researchers involved with developing case definitions for CMI in 1990–1991 Gulf War Veterans.
- Discussions with clinicians who treat Veterans of the 1990-1991 Gulf War.

In addition to reviewing and summarizing the available scientific and medical literature regarding symptoms and case definitions for CMI among Gulf War Veterans, the committee will:

- Establish a consensus case definition along with guidelines for its use.
- Evaluate existing case definitions in relation to priorities identified by the committee and determine whether an existing case definition is adequate, an existing case definition needs to be revised, or a new case definition needs to be established.
- Consider issues such as specificity (the degree to which the definition applies to 1990–1991 Gulf War Veterans), sensitivity (the degree to which the case definition captures the excess symptomatology in 1990–1991 Gulf War Veterans), reliability (the degree to which Veterans' symptoms are determined in a consistent manner), and portability (the degree to which the case definition is suitable for use in different study designs) in evaluating case definitions.5
- Consider the potential for the case definition, optimized for research purposes, to be used in clinical practice.
- Consider other case definition characteristics deemed important.
- Recommend additional areas of research or study that may be required to more adequately develop a consensus definition for CMI in 1990–1991 Gulf War Veterans.
- Evaluate the terminology currently used in referring to CMI in Gulf War Veterans and recommend appropriate usage.

---

[4]The committee uses the term *chronic multisymptom illness* throughout the report, as defined in the statement of work, when referring to the symptom complex in Gulf War veterans.
[5]In completing its analysis, the committee clarified the definitions of sensitivity and specificity in Chapter 2.

HOW THE COMMITTEE APPROACHED ITS CHARGE

The IOM appointed a committee of 16 experts to carry out the task. The committee members have expertise in occupational medicine, biostatistics, psychometrics, epidemiology, basic science, clinical medicine, toxicology, psychiatry, neurology, gastroenterology, and sociology. Some of the committee members treated Gulf War veterans when they came to their clinics or practices, and one committee members' practice is devoted solely to Gulf War and other veterans. The committee also consulted with an expert in brain imaging because that field was not represented on the committee.

The committee members directed the staff to conduct an extensive search of the extant peer-reviewed literature. PubMed was searched for all references related to the 1990–1991 Gulf War. Initially, more than 5,000 papers were retrieved; after elimination of duplicates, 2,033 unique papers remained. The titles and abstracts of those papers were reviewed, and 718 were selected for more rigorous review. The committee members divided the work by reading papers related to their expertise. The papers that were reviewed included all health outcomes that have been noted in Gulf War veterans, for example, mortality, hospitalization, neurologic symptoms, respiratory symptoms, gastrointestinal symptoms, pain, birth defects and fertility, cancer, mental-health conditions, and overlapping syndromes. In an effort to characterize the symptomatology associated with CMI, the focus of the committee's review is on studies of symptoms not associated with diagnosed medical or psychiatric conditions; the focus is on studies of symptom-reporting in Gulf War veterans. The committee agreed early on that a determination of the etiology of CMI was outside the scope of its charge. Thus, the committee did not consider toxicologic or exposure studies.

The committee held one open meeting, in which members heard from veterans, government officials, researchers, clinicians who treat Gulf War veterans, and members of the VA Research Advisory Committee. The meeting increased the committee's awareness of the variety of symptoms being experienced by the Gulf War veterans. In addition, the vigorous discussions with the veterans and researchers were invaluable for increasing the committee members' understanding of the complexity of issues involved in its task.

ORGANIZATION OF THE REPORT

Chapter 2 introduces some of the issues that have made CMI so difficult to define and presents the general elements of case definitions. Chapter 3 summarizes the many cohort studies that focus on the Gulf War veterans' symptomatology. It discusses how the cohorts were assembled, the limitations of the studies, and the array of symptoms identified. Chapter 4 provides a brief discussion of factor analysis and discusses previous efforts related to the use of factor analyses to detect a unique syndrome in Gulf War veterans. Finally, Chapter 5 presents the committee's discussion of existing case definitions of CMI and its conclusions and recommendations. The report has two appendixes: Appendix A contains additional background information on statistical techniques used to identify a unique Gulf War syndrome, and Appendix B contains a graph depicting the range of percentages of symptoms endorsed by veterans.

REFERENCES

Brown, M. 2006. Toxicological assessments of Gulf War veterans. *Philosophical transactions of the Royal Society of London. Series B, Biological Sciences* 361(1468):649-679.

DOD (Department of Defense). 1992. *TRADOC Support to Operations Desert Shield and Desert Storm: A Preliminary Study.* Office of the Command Historian, US Army Training and Doctrine Command.

GAO (Government Accounting Office). 2004. *Gulf War Illnesses: DOD's Conclusions about U.S. Troops' Exposure Cannot Be Adequately Supported.* Washington, DC: US Government Accountability Office.

IOM (Institute of Medicine). 2000. *Gulf War and Health, Volume 1: Depleted Uranium, Pyrodostigmine Bromide, Sarin, Vaccines*. Washington, DC: National Academy Press.

IOM. 2003. *Gulf War and Health, Volume 2: Insecticides and Solvents*. Washington, DC: The National Academies Press.

IOM. 2005. *Gulf War and Health, Volume 3: Fuels, Combustion Products, and Propellants*. Washington, DC: The National Academies Press.

Joseph, S. C., R. R. Blanck, G. Gackstetter, R. Glaser, K. C. Hyams, S. Kinty, C. Magruder, J. Mazzuchi, F. L. O'Donnell, M. D. Parkinson, R. E. Patterson, and D. H. Trump. 1997. A comprehensive clinical evaluation of 20,000 Persian Gulf War veterans. *Military Medicine* 162(3):149-155.

King's College London. 2010. *King's Centre for Military Health Research: A Fifteen Year Report. What Has Been Achieved by Fifteen Years of Research into the Health of the UK Armed Forces?* University of London.

2

CASE DEFINITIONS

This chapter considers some of the challenges in defining chronic multisymptom illness (CMI), including the array of symptoms experienced by Gulf War veterans, the absence of a clear etiology, the sparseness of data on onset or illness duration, the lack of diagnostic tests, and the many names and methods by which this illness has been characterized. It then focuses on the general elements of a case definition and examines case definitions of other symptom-based disorders.

ADDRESSING CHRONIC MULTISYMPTOM ILLNESS IN GULF WAR VETERANS

Although many Gulf War veterans suffer from an array of health problems and symptoms (such as fatigue, muscle and joint pain, memory loss, and gastrointestinal disorders), those health issues are not necessarily peculiar to any identified disease and are not satisfactorily classified by standard diagnostic coding systems (IOM, 2010). Population-based studies have found a higher prevalence of symptom reporting in Gulf War veterans than in nondeployed Gulf War era veterans or other control groups (Goss Gilroy Inc., 1998; Iowa Persian Gulf Study Group, 1997; Unwin et al., 1999), as discussed in Chapter 3. The wide variation in symptoms reported by Gulf War veterans has complicated efforts to determine whether there is a unique Gulf War syndrome or whether symptom patterns are more consistent with other known symptom-based disorders. Consequently, the array of symptoms suffered by many Gulf War veterans does not often point to an obvious diagnosis, etiology, or specific treatment.

The search for a definitive cause of CMI also has been difficult. The veterans of the 1990–1991 Gulf War were exposed to an impressive array of biologic and chemical agents, as noted in Chapter 1. Numerous studies have been conducted over the past 20 years to determine an etiology based on exposure to many substances, such as pyridostigmine bromide (PB), anthrax vaccine, tent-heater fumes, oil-fire smoke, and chemical odors (Wolfe et al., 2002); jet fuel (Bell et al., 2005); sarin and cyclosarin (Chao et al., 2011); and combinations of organophosphate pesticides, chemical nerve agents, DEET insect repellent, and PB (Haley and Kurt, 1997; Haley et al., 1999). However, exposures during the Gulf War were not reliably measured (if they were measured at all), and most often exposure has been evaluated through surveys or health examinations some years after it occurred (Gray et al., 2004). The association between retrospective recall of exposures and self-reported health outcomes is subject to recall bias (discussed in Chapter 3). No coherent mechanism of action or definitive causal association between the exposures and the range of symptoms reported has been established (Barrett et al., 2002).

Even the terminology used over the years has at times been perplexing. Initially, the term *Gulf War syndrome* was used; numerous other terms—such as *Gulf War illness*, *unexplained illness*, *medically unexplained symptoms* or *medically unexplained physical symptoms*, and *chronic multisymptom illness*—appeared in the medical and scientific literature. Many of the symptoms of CMI overlap with those of other diseases and ill-defined conditions, such as fibromyalgia (FM) and chronic fatigue syndrome (CFS). As noted by Ismail and Lewis (2006), when several symptoms are reported together in the absence of evidence of a physical cause, they are often termed medically unexplained syndromes. It adds to the difficulty of defining CMI and finding a common etiology that the literature contains a number of discussions that refer to different postwar syndromes (see Table 2.1) as possible explanations of the illnesses in Gulf War veterans (e.g., Engel, 2004; Hyams et al., 1996).

Many similarities between previously identified postwar syndromes and CMI have been noted. More generally, all modern wars have been associated with medically unexplained symptoms or syndromes (Jones et al., 2002). Thus, if military personnel are deployed to war zones, some of those returning will have such illnesses. For instance, a systematic comparison of UK pension files from previous wars (the Boer War, World War I, and World War II) with clinical files from the Gulf War, revealed that CMI is similar to many postconflict syndromes. During the Boer War, soldiers complained primarily of fatigue, rheumatic pains, weakness, shortness of breath, rapid heart rate, headache, and dizziness. In World Wars I and II, primary symptom complaints were chest pain, breathlessness, dizziness, and fatigue and to a lesser extent headache and anxiety (King's College London, 2010).

TABLE 2.1 Postwar Illnesses

War	Syndrome or Illness
US Civil War	Da Costa syndrome, irritable heart syndrome
World War I	Soldier's heart or the effort syndrome
World War II	Acute combat stress reaction, battle fatigue, combat exhaustion
Korean Conflict	Acute combat stress reaction
Vietnam War	Post-Vietnam syndrome, posttraumatic stress disorder

With regard to specific symptoms reported by the veterans of the 1990–1991 Gulf War, numerous studies have been conducted and details of the symptoms reported. The studies have been summarized and evaluated by previous Institute of Medicine committees (IOM, 2006, 2010), and many are discussed in Chapters 3 and 4 of the present report. A 10-year followup study that tracked the health of 1990–1991 Gulf War veterans found that deployed veterans continued to report persistently poorer health than nondeployed veterans (Li et al., 2011). It was also found that the deployed veterans were less likely to improve and more likely to experience a new onset of adverse health outcomes, including fatigue, than their nondeployed counterparts. In brief, the studies showed that symptom reporting was inconsistent among studies and that no single symptom complex, or syndrome, was identified. However, deployed 1990–1991 Gulf War veterans reported a higher prevalence of fatigue, nervous system symptoms, respiratory symptoms, chronic musculoskeletal pain, gastrointestinal symptoms, mood and cognitive abnormalities, and sleep disturbance than did nondeployed 1991 Gulf War–era veterans.

Furthermore, estimates of the prevalence of CMI among deployed 1991 Gulf War veterans vary widely by study population (see Chapter 3).

DEVELOPING CASE DEFINITIONS

In the United States, state and local health officials are required by state laws or regulations to report some diseases. Having standard case definitions for reportable diseases is critical for physicians, health care providers, and other health officials so that they can provide local and federal organizations with information about outbreaks, poisonings, and so on. And having criteria for accurate diagnosis of particular diseases or conditions enables health care providers to prescribe standard treatments. It enables researchers to enroll patients into research and drug trials that are aimed at bringing about cures or treatments. Having defined case definitions also enhances the search for commonalities among cases in an effort to identify causative agents.

According to the Centers for Disease Control and Prevention (CDC), case definitions, particularly related to outbreaks, include criteria associated with persons, places, times, and clinical features (see Table 2.2). Case definitions are important for standardizing criteria for identification of cases.

TABLE 2.2 Elements of a Case Definition

Element	Descriptive Feature
Person	Age Sex Occupation Exclusion criteria Race
Place	Geographic location
Time	Illness onset
Clinical features	Depend on the condition to be defined
Laboratory criteria	Blood tests, imaging, and so on

SOURCE: Adapted from CDC, 2008.

A case definition may include criteria that can be used effectively to identify a patient population and distinguish it from patient populations that have similar recognized diagnoses. Case definitions may be derived through clinical evaluation. Clinically derived case definitions are usually formulated a priori by investigators on the basis of commonly reported symptoms. The development of a first case definition may be more like a hypothesis than a conclusion; it is an early step in the process of identifying a new clinical entity and depends on further research. Case definitions commonly change as new evidence becomes available.

Issues of sensitivity and specificity arise in case definitions. A sensitive case definition might be broad in its reach in an effort to capture all people who have the disease but may inadvertently capture some who do not have the disease, whereas a more specific definition might be too narrow and include only people who have the disease but will probably miss some cases. Therefore, case definitions are often adapted for different uses. For example, for particular research purposes, a sample with high positive predictive value might be desirable; that is, a pure sample in which all the subjects who are called cases have a very high probability of actually being cases. For physicians, the primary purposes of a consensus case definition may be to serve as the basis for determining appropriate clinical approaches to evaluation and treatment of those who are affected and to inform the natural history of the condition so that it may be studied (Wegman et al., 1997).

Case Definitions of Symptom-Based Disorders

It is not unusual for some disorders and syndromes not to have an agreed-on case definition or to have multiple case definitions. It is difficult to identify cases in the absence of confirmatory physical signs or laboratory findings and without a known etiology or pathophysiology. The use of case-definition criteria to identify symptoms and validate many serious disorders, such as irritable bowel syndrome (IBS), has been difficult, frustrating, costly, and time-consuming for clinicians, patients, family members, and caretakers. Often, the first attempts at classifying the symptoms for a case definition are not widely accepted—for example, the Manning criteria for IBS followed by the Rome criteria in 1988 (*Rome III: The Functional Gastrointestinal Disorders*, 2006; Talley et al., 1990). The criteria must be validated to assess their usefulness in clinical and research settings. In many instances, diagnosis of symptom-based conditions requires the exclusion of other conditions, and this may place a serious burden on the patient and the health care system. In addition, symptom-based criteria may be used inappropriately and might be limited to specific populations (Yale et al., 2008).

The case definitions of chronic fatigue syndrome (CFS) have met with similar problems. For the past 25 years, a wealth of information regarding myalgic encephalomyelitis (ME) and CFS (ME/CFS) has been accumulated. Despite the progress, however, there is still no accurate diagnostic test or proven treatment. Like *chronic multisymptom illness*, the term *chronic fatigue syndrome* has been criticized as being vague and trivializing the illness. A number of overlapping case definitions have been published; however, the great majority of research studies use the CDC definition of CFS[1] (Fukuda et al., 1994). Like the diagnosis of CMI, the diagnosis of CFS is based on patient-reported symptoms; there is no validated diagnostic test. The diagnosis of ME/CFS is based on the patient's history, the pattern of symptoms, and the exclusion of other fatiguing illnesses. A symptom-based diagnosis can be made on the basis of published criteria. The 2003 Canadian clinical case definition of ME/CFS (Carruthers et al., 2003) and the 2011 international clinical criteria for ME (Carruthers et al., 2011) are intended to emphasize clearly described core symptoms of the illness. The 1994 Fukuda criteria for CFS are used primarily for research purposes, however, they may be used clinically, and may be required for disability determinations in the United States and elsewhere.

Like CMI and many other symptom-based illnesses, ME/CFS is not without controversy, particularly regarding whether they are mental disorders or physical health disorders (IACFSME, 2012). The committee notes that this either/or approach is not useful, for several reasons. The distinction between mental and physical disorders is often arbitrary, and most patients' experiences of any illness are influenced by biologic, psychologic, and social factors. Either/or thinking leads too often to a presumption that medically unexplained symptoms must be psychogenic. In addition, psychiatric symptoms may not be fully evaluated if a patient's symptoms are psychogenic. Although physical and psychologic stress can exacerbate many chronic conditions—including chronic pain, headache, respiratory, and gastrointestinal

---

[1] CDC was the first agency to define CFS.

symptoms—there is an inherent risk in assuming that medically unexplained symptoms assume a "stress-induced" etiology. Nearly one-third of physical symptoms presenting in primary care are psychiatric or medically unexplained (Kroenke and Price, 1993). There has been a tendency to dismiss medically unexplained symptoms, but they are disabling and associated with poor quality of life (Ismail and Lewis, 2006).

Case Definitions of Chronic Multisymptom Illness in Gulf War Veterans

One of the tasks of the committee was to examine the peer-reviewed literature specific to deployed Gulf War veterans' symptomatology in an effort to develop or identify a case definition that will show adequate sensitivity and specificity for research and treatment purposes. In the numerous symptom studies reviewed by the committee, the array of symptoms reported makes it difficult to identify hallmark characteristics of the illness. In addition, the symptoms detailed in Gulf War veterans are shared by other symptom-based disorders, such as CFS and FM, and are seen in the general adult population. There are no objective diagnostic criteria, such as laboratory abnormalities or characteristic physical signs, so diagnosing symptom-based conditions, such as CMI, often must depend on the exclusion of other causes. Thus, specificity becomes a major limitation in developing a case definition of CMI. As noted by Hyams (1998), specificity requires a low proportion of false positives; however, without diagnostic criteria that exclude well-recognized medical and psychiatric causes of symptoms and distinguish them from other symptom-based conditions, a specific diagnosis has not been possible.

Studies that do present a case definition of CMI do not often satisfy the criteria required for a case definition as described above. Although researchers can identify the exposed population (the 1990–1991 Gulf War veterans), it is difficult to assign uniform clinical criteria to all suspected cases or to know the exact time of onset, the duration and severity of symptoms, and so on. Thus, case definitions of symptom-based disorders are often difficult to develop and require continued attention and adjustment as new information becomes available.

REFERENCES

Barrett, D. H., G. C. Gray, B. N. Doebbeling, D. J. Clauw, and W. C. Reeves. 2002. Prevalence of symptoms and symptom-based conditions among Gulf War veterans: Current status of research findings. *Epidemiologic Reviews* 24(2):218-227.

Bell, I. R., A. J. Brooks, C. M. Baldwin, M. Fernandez, A. J. Figueredo, and M. L. Witten. 2005. JP-8 jet fuel exposure and divided attention test performance in 1991 Gulf War veterans. *Aviation Space and Environmental Medicine* 76(12):1136-1144.

Blanchard, M. S., S. A. Eisen, R. Alpern, J. Karlinsky, R. Toomey, D. J. Reda, F. M. Murphy, L. W. Jackson, and H. K. Kang. 2006. Chronic multisymptom illness complex in Gulf War I veterans 10 years later. *American Journal of Epidemiology* 163(1):66-75.

Carruthers, B. M., M. I. van de Sande, K. L. De Meirleir, N. G. Klimas, G. Broderick, T. Mitchell, D. Staines, A. C. Powles, N. Speight, R. Vallings, L. Bateman, B. Baumgarten-Austrheim, D. S. Bell, N. Carlo-Stella, J. Chia, A. Darragh, D. Jo, D. Lewis, A. R. Light, S. Marshall-Gradisbik, I. Mena, J. A. Mikovits, K. Miwa, M. Murovska, M. L. Pall, and S. Stevens. 2011. Myalgic encephalomyelitis: International consensus criteria. *Journal of Internal Medicine* 270(4):327-338.

CDC (Centers for Disease Control and Prevention). 2008. *Outbreak Case Definitions*. http://emergency.cdc.gov/urdo/pdf/CaseDefinitions.pdf (accessed August 8, 2013).

Chao, L. L., L. Abadjian, J. Hlavin, D. J. Meyerhoff, and M. W. Weiner. 2011. Effects of low-level sarin and cyclosarin exposure and Gulf War illness on brain structure and function: A study at 4T. *Neurotoxicology* 32(6):814-822.

Engel, C. C., Jr. 2004. Post-war syndromes: Illustrating the impact of the social psyche on notions of risk, responsibility, reason, and remedy. *Journal of the American Academy of Psychoanalysis and Dynamic Psychiatry* 32(2):321-334; discussion 335-343.

Fukuda, K., S. E. Straus, I. Hickie, M. C. Sharpe, J. G. Dobbins, and A. Komaroff. 1994. The chronic fatigue syndrome: A comprehensive approach to its definition and study. International Chronic Fatigue Syndrome Study Group. *Annals of Internal Medicine* 121(12):953-959.

Fukuda, K., R. Nisenbaum, G. Stewart, W. W. Thompson, L. Robin, R. M. Washko, D. L. Noah, D. H. Barrett, B. Randall, B. L. Herwaldt, A. C. Mawle, and W. C. Reeves. 1998. Chronic multisymptom illness affecting Air Force veterans of the Gulf War. *Journal of the American Medical Association* 280(11):981-988.

Goss Gilroy Inc. 1998. Health Study of Canadian Forces Personnel Involved in the 1991 Conflict in the Persian Gulf. Ottawa, Canada: Goss Gilroy Inc. Department of National Defence.

Gray, G. C., G. D. Gackstetter, H. K. Kang, J. T. Graham, and K. C. Scott. 2004. After more than 10 years of Gulf War veteran medical evaluations, what have we learned? *American Journal of Preventive Medicine* 26(5):443-452.

Haley, R. W., and T. L. Kurt. 1997. Self-reported exposure to neurotoxic chemical combinations in the Gulf War: A cross-sectional epidemiologic study. *Journal of the American Medical Association* 277(3):231-237.

Haley, R. W., S. Billecke, and B. N. La Du. 1999. Association of low PON1 type Q (type A) arylesterase activity with neurologic symptom complexes in Gulf War veterans. *Toxicology and Applied Pharmacology* 157(3):227-233.

Hyams, K. C. 1998. Developing case definitions for symptom-based conditions: The problem of specificity. *Epidemiologic Reviews* 20(2):148-156.

Hyams, K. C., F. S. Wignall, and R. Roswell. 1996. War Syndromes and Their Evaluation: From the U.S. Civil War to the Persian Gulf War. *Annals of Internal Medicine* 125(5):398-405.

IACFSME (International Association for Chronic Fatigue Syndrome/Myalgic Encephalomyelitis). 2012. *ME/CFS: A Primer for Clinical Practioners*. www.iacfsme.org/portals/0/pdf/primerfinal3.pdf (accessed August 8, 2013).

IOM (Institute of Medicine). 2006. *Gulf War and Health, Volume 4: Health Effects of Serving in the Gulf War*. Washington, DC: The National Academies Press.

IOM. 2010. *Gulf War and Health, Volume 8: Update of Health Effects of Serving in the Gulf War*. Washington, DC: The National Academies Press.

Iowa Persian Gulf Study Group. 1997. Self-reported illness and health status among Gulf War veterans: A population-based study. *Journal of the American Medical Association* 277(3):238-245.

Ismail, K., and G. Lewis. 2006. Multi-symptom illnesses, unexplained illness and Gulf War Syndrome. *Philosophical Transactions of the Royal Society B: Biological Sciences* 361(1468):543-551.

Jones, E., R. Hodgins-Vermaas, H. McCartney, B. Everitt, C. Beech, D. Poynter, I. Palmer, K. Hyams, and S. Wessely. 2002. Post-combat syndromes from the Boer War to the Gulf War: A cluster analysis of their nature and attribution. *British Medical Journal* 324(7333):321-324.

King's College London. 2010. *King's Centre for Military Health Research: A Fifteen Year Report. What Has Been Achieved by Fifteen Years of Research into the Health of the UK Armed Forces?* University of London.

Kroenke, K., and R. Price. 1993. Symptoms in the community: Prevalence, classification and psychiatric comorbidity. *Archives of Internal Medicine* 153:2474–2480.

Li, B., C. M. Mahan, H. K. Kang, S. A. Eisen, and C. C. Engel. 2011. Longitudinal health study of US 1991 Gulf War veterans: Changes in health status at 10-year follow-up. *American Journal of Epidemiology* 174(7):761-768.

Rome III: The Functional Gastrointestinal Disorders. 2006. Edited by D. A. Drossman. Vol. 3: Rome Foundation.

Talley, N. J., S. F. Phillips, L. J. Melton, C. Mulvihill, C. Wiltgen, and A. R. Zinsmeister. 1990. Diagnostic value of the Manning criteria in irritable bowel syndrome. *Gut* 31(1):77-81.

Unwin, C., N. Blatchley, W. Coker, S. Ferry, M. Hotopf, L. Hull, K. Ismail, I. Palmer, A. David, and S. Wessely. 1999. Health of UK servicemen who served in Persian Gulf War. *Lancet* 353(9148):169-178.

Wegman, D. H., N. F. Woods, and J. C. Bailar. 1997. Invited commentary: How would we know a Gulf War syndrome if we saw one? *American Journal of Epidemiology* 146(9):704-711; discussion 712.

Wolfe, J., S. P. Proctor, D. J. Erickson, and H. Hu. 2002. Risk Factors for Multisymptom Illness in US Army Veterans of the Gulf War. *Journal of Occupational and Environmental Medicine* 44(3):271-281.

Yale, S. H., A. K. Musana, A. Kieke, J. Hayes, I. Glurich, and P. H. Chyou. 2008. Applying case definition criteria to irritable bowel syndrome. *Clinical Medicine & Research* 6(1):9-16.

3

STUDIES OF SYMPTOMS IN GULF WAR VETERANS

This chapter provides an overview of the cohorts that were assembled to study the symptoms of the 1990–1991 Gulf War veterans. It discusses the limitations of the studies and summarizes the finding of each. Some of the cohorts were brought together in the first few years after the Gulf War; others were assembled later. Most of the studies compare sizable groups of deployed veterans with groups of veterans who were not deployed during the period of the Gulf War (often referred to as era veterans) or who were deployed to locations other than the Persian Gulf (for example, Bosnia) during the period (referred to as deployed elsewhere). In addition, a number of volunteer registries were assembled by the US Department of Defense (DOD) and Department of Veterans Affairs (VA) and by other governments whose forces were included in the Gulf War coalition. All those groups constitute the major cohorts that are described in this chapter.

The chapter's focus on symptom studies, rather than on studies of well-characterized diagnosed medical and psychiatric conditions, provides the foundation for the committee's understanding of the symptomatology experienced by the Gulf War veterans. Some of the authors have conducted factor analyses or proposed case definitions, and those studies are discussed in Chapters 4 and 5.

The chapter begins with a discussion of the limitations seen throughout the studies, which is followed by a description of the cohorts assembled after the Gulf War. The studies detail the symptoms found in the Gulf War veterans. They are organized by a key feature of the studies' design: how the study populations were defined. Three categories of studies were identified—population-based, military unit–based, and registry-based. The discussion of each study includes a summary of its methods and its major findings pertaining to reported symptoms. Table 3.1, summarizing all the studies reviewed, is at the end of the chapter.

GENERAL LIMITATIONS OF GULF WAR STUDIES

The cohort studies of Gulf War veterans and their derivatives have contributed greatly to our understanding of veterans' health but are subject to limitations that are commonly encountered in observational epidemiologic studies. They include selection biases that limit the studies' representativeness and generalizability to the larger veteran population; self-reporting of health outcomes and exposures, which is affected by recall bias; outcome misclassification; and reporting bias.[1] Box 3.1 briefly summarizes some of the general biases that affect this body of literature.

Bias refers to the systematic, or nonrandom, tendency for an observed value to deviate from a true value because of flaws in study design and methods. A biased design may result in weakening an association, in strengthening an association, or in generating a spurious association. Because all studies are susceptible to bias, a primary goal of research design is to minimize bias or to adjust the observed value of an association by correcting for bias if its sources are known.

There are two major types of bias: *selection bias* and *information bias*. Selection bias involves a systematic error—in how subjects are identified, recruited, included, or excluded or in how they participate in a study—that leads to a distortion of a true association. Information bias results from how data are collected and can result in measurement errors, imprecise measurement, and misclassification. Those biases may be uniform in an entire study population or may affect some subgroups of the population more than others.

BOX 3.1
Common Medical-Research Biases That Affect Studies of Gulf War and Health

Selection bias: Bias can result from selection of participants in such a way that they do not represent the target population or the probability of selection is related to exposure or disease status. This may be due to a poor definition of the eligible population or failure to obtain a random sample. Includes

Nonresponse bias: Participants have a different exposure or disease status from nonparticipants.

Volunteer bias: Participants who volunteer are more likely to have the exposure or disease of interest; this is a particular problem for registry studies that collect information on participants who enroll voluntarily.

Healthy-warrior effect: Veterans or personnel who were deployed may be healthier than those who were not deployed or than civilians; selection of healthier people occurs at enlistment and separation (ill and injured personnel are more likely to leave the military).

Information or measurement bias: Misclassification of participants' exposure or disease status may be based on the information collected by various methods (such as a mailed questionnaire, a telephone interview, record review, or a medical examination). Includes

Recall bias: The presence of disease influences participants' reflection and perception of possible causes and can make them likely to report more exposures than or different exposures from nondiseased participants.

Reporting bias: Participants are more likely to report responses that they perceive as favorable and to underreport undesirable responses.

Temporal ambiguity: This occurs when it cannot be established that an exposure occurred before the onset of disease; it is common in cross-sectional assessments.

Confounding: This occurs when a risk factor for the disease that is also related to the exposure creates a spurious exposure–disease association; in other words, a risk factor may cause the exposed and nonexposed participants to have different background disease risks.

SOURCES: Delgado-Rodríguez and Llorca, 2004; Levenson et al., 1990; Pearce et al., 2006.

[1]Biases previously described by the IOM (2006, 2010).

An important limitation is selection bias, which results in a lack of representativeness and limits one's ability to generalize results to the entire population of interest; this is related to what is known as external validity. For example, six of the cohorts are made up of veterans that were selected according to where they served in the military (a military unit–based study) (Fukuda et al., 1998; Gray et al., 1999; Haley et al., 1997; Pierce, 1997; Proctor et al., 1998; Stretch et al., 1995). Military-unit studies are not representative of all Gulf War veterans with respect to their duties and locations during deployment, possible exposures, military status during the war (active duty, reserves, or National Guard), military status after the war (active duty, reserves, or discharged), branch of service (Army, Navy, Air Force, or Marine Corps), or ease of ascertainment (IOM, 1999).

In population-based cohort studies, a sample or the entire defined population is selected for longitudinal study. Ideally, a population-based study starts prospectively with a cohort that is convened before the exposure or onset of symptoms. The study of a cohort, that is representative of a defined population offers several advantages. For example, it allows the estimation of distributions and prevalences of relevant variables in the reference population; risk-factor distributions measured at baseline in a study involving periodic examinations of the cohort can be compared with distributions in future cross-sectional samples to assess risk-factor trends over time; and a representative sample is the ideal setting in which to carry out unbiased evaluations of relationships not only of confounders to exposures and outcomes but also among any other variables of interest (Szklo, 1998).

Some population-based studies of Gulf War veterans sample a cohort of veterans by contacting them where they live as opposed to where they seek treatment or where they serve in the military (for example, a particular base or a particular branch, such as the Air Force). Studies of military units or other military groups are less representative of the broader Gulf War veteran population than are population-based studies. Military unit–based studies are generalizable only to members of that unit and not to the broader veteran or military population Large population-based studies of Gulf War veterans have been conducted in each of the three major countries that participated in the Gulf War coalition: the United States, Canada, and the United Kingdom (Cherry et al., 2001; Goss Gilroy Inc., 1998; Kang et al., 2000; Unwin et al., 1999).

Representativeness is also compromised when some demographic groups are underrepresented in the study sample, such as women. Some studies used methods to increase a sample's representativeness by oversampling specific groups. For example, Kang et al. (2000) oversampled women and those serving in the National Guard and reserves, and this resulted in a study sample that was about 20% women, 25% National Guard, and 33% reservists. The controls were stratified by sex, unit, and branch of service to mirror the population of deployed veterans.

A study's representativeness, even if it is population-based, can be compromised by low participation or response rates, which may result in *nonresponse bias*. For example, Gulf War veterans who are symptomatic may choose to participate more frequently than those who are not symptomatic. Response rates in the studies discussed in this chapter are highly variable; they range from 92% (Steele, 2000; Wolfe et al., 1998) to 28% (Salamon et al., 2006). In some studies, researchers not only try to measure nonresponse bias by comparing participants with nonparticipants from both deployed and nondeployed populations but make adjustments to overcome it, for example, by oversampling nondeployed populations.

Quite different from population-based studies are ones that rely on voluntary participants to identify themselves, such as those who volunteer to participate in a registry. Registry studies may be subject to *volunteer bias*. They should be interpreted with caution inasmuch as registry participants are self-selected (sicker people are more likely to join) and not representative of the entire Gulf War veteran population. In addition, they often do not include a control group for comparison.

Selection bias might also occur through the so-called *healthy-warrior effect*. That bias has the potential to occur in most of the major cohorts that compare deployed veterans with nondeployed personnel. The healthy-warrior effect is a form of selection bias in that chronically ill or less fit members of the armed forces might be less likely to have been deployed than more fit members. That is, there might have been nonrandom assignment of those selected and not selected for deployment.

Some studies attempt to measure the potential for selection bias and adjust for it in the analysis. Other studies compare Gulf War deployed veterans with two or more groups, such as veterans deployed to other locations or missions (Hotopf and Wessely, 2005).

Many issues can contribute to information bias or measurement bias and result in the misclassification of people as sick or healthy when they are not. Symptom self-reporting might sometimes introduce *outcome misclassification*, in which there are errors in how symptoms are classified into outcomes and analyzed. One Gulf War study sought to document outcome misclassification by comparing veterans' symptom reporting on questionnaires with results of clinical examination about 3 months later (McCauley et al., 1999). The authors found that the extent of misclassification depended on the type of symptom being reported; agreement between questionnaire and clinical examination ranged from 4% to 79%. The overall problem led the investigators to caution that questionnaire data, in the absence of clinical evaluation or adjustment, might lead to outcome misclassification. Another study also found poor reliability and validity of self-reported diagnoses compared with medical records (Gray et al., 1999). In contrast, a study by VA (Kang et al., 2000), which verified a random subset of self-reported conditions against medical records, found a strong correlation between the two (above 93%). Those data, however, were available only for the 45.2% who signed consent forms that allowed researchers to verify records.

Another important limitation is that most cohort studies rely on self-reporting of symptoms on questionnaires. Most of the larger epidemiologic studies described here were conducted through mail or telephone surveys, and this precluded clinical examination and diagnosis. Studies based on self-reporting have inherent limitations because of potential inaccuracies in recalling past events and difficulty in verifying the reports. Symptom self-reporting potentially introduces *reporting bias*, which occurs when the group being studied (such as deployed veterans) overreports particular symptoms (such as symptoms that are more intense or more recently experienced), that is, reports the symptoms more frequently than a comparison group (such as nondeployed veterans). Reporting bias, in this example, would lead to an overestimation of the prevalence of symptoms or diagnoses in the deployed population. Similarly, self-reporting of exposures is problematic and subject to *recall bias* in that sick soldiers may be more likely to report that they were exposed. Issues arising as a result of symptom self-reporting are best addressed through clinical evaluations, as has been done by some researchers (Ishøy et al., 1999a; Kelsall et al., 2005; McCauley et al., 1999). Many limitations of reporting and recall bias are present in Gulf War research (e.g., Murphy et al., 2006, 2008).

Virtually all the studies cited in this chapter are cross-sectional—surveys, questionnaires, interviews, and the like were conducted at a single time—and can thus be subject to *temporal ambiguity*. Even though some studies conduct serial cross-sectional assessments over time (Kang et al., 2000, 2009), the timing of retrospective exposures and symptoms is difficult to ascertain, and this limits the opportunity to learn about symptom duration and chronicity, latency of onset, prognosis, and potential causal factors.

Many other factors can affect the association between an exposure and an outcome, including lifestyle, hereditary factors, and additional exposures, which are known as *confounding* factors. Confounding occurs when a variable or characteristic otherwise known to be predictive of an outcome and associated with an exposure (and not on the causal pathway under consideration) can account for all or part of an apparent association. A confounding variable is an uncontrolled variable that influences the outcome of a study to an unknown extent and whose effects cannot be precisely evaluated. Carefully applied statistical adjustments can often control for or reduce the influence of a confounder (IOM, 2010).

Other limitations of the body of evidence are that studies might be too narrow in their assessment of health status, the measurement instruments might have been too insensitive to detect abnormalities that affect deployed veterans, and the period of investigation might have been too brief to detect health outcomes that have a long latency or require many years to progress to disability, hospitalization, or death. Finally, research into the health effects of Gulf War deployment is limited by the interval between the war and when the studies were conducted. Many studies were conducted years after the war, and this limits the ability to determine when symptoms developed and the ability to detect causal associations—for example, the earliest assessments were conducted in 1993 by Pierce (1997) and Wolfe et al. (1998), in 1994 by Gray et al. (1999), and in 1995 by Fukuda et al. (1998). Followup of the cohorts is also limited because some active military separate each year. And the delay between the war and the studies allows the dissemination of speculation by the media and others that may have affected veterans' recall (Hotopf and Wessely, 2005).

POPULATION-BASED STUDIES

The following are population-based studies of samples of veterans or military personnel. VA conducted a nationally representative study of Gulf War veterans (Kang et al., 2000, 2002, 2009). Several studies of selected population-based samples of veterans defined by state of residence were conducted (Bourdette et al., 2001; Iowa Persian Gulf Study Group, 1997; McCauley et al., 1999; Steele, 2000). Finally, several additional studies of populations of allied military personnel are described (Cherry et al., 2001; Goss Gilroy Inc., 1998; Hotopf and Wessely, 2005; Ishøy et al., 1999a; Kelsall et al., 2004; Simmons et al., 2004; Unwin et al., 1999).

Department of Veterans Affairs Study

VA conducted a study that used the National Health Survey of Gulf War Veterans and Their Families to estimate the prevalence of symptoms and other health outcomes (including reproductive outcomes in spouses and birth defects in children) in Gulf War veterans vs nondeployed Gulf War–era veterans. The three-phase retrospective study was designed to be representative of nearly 700,000 US veterans who were deployed to the Persian Gulf and 800,680 veterans who were not deployed but were in the military during September 1990–May 1991. In the first phase, questionnaires were mailed to 30,000 veterans (15,000 Gulf War deployed and 15,000 era veterans) identified by the DOD Data Manpower Center as representing the various branches and units of the military. The questionnaire contained a list of 48 symptoms and questions about chronic medical conditions, functional limitations, and other items from the National Health Interview Survey and included questions about exposures. The overall response rate was about 70%. The second phase used telephone interview software in an attempt to capture those who did not respond to the mailed questionnaires. In addition, medical records were obtained for a random sample of 4,200 respondents to validate self-reports of clinic visits or hospitalizations within the preceding year. The third phase was a comprehensive medical examination, including laboratory testing, of a random sample of 2,000 veterans drawn from the Gulf War population and a comparison group (Kang et al., 2000).

The investigation found that Gulf War veterans reported statistically significantly greater functional impairment in the preceding 2 weeks (27.8% vs 14.2%), limitation of employment (17.2% vs 11.6%), and health care use in the preceding year as assessed on the basis of clinic visits (50.8% vs 40.5%) and hospitalizations (7.8% vs 6.4%) than era veterans. Gulf War veterans reported higher prevalences of all 48 symptoms on the health inventory. The most frequently reported were runny nose, headache, unrefreshing sleep, anxiety, joint pain, back pain, fatigue, ringing in ears, heartburn, difficulty in sleeping, depression, and difficulty in concentrating (see Table 3.2) (Kang et al. 2000). Those 12 symptoms are similar in prevalence to the same symptoms in a UK cohort (Unwin et al., 1999). In a randomly selected subset of veterans, medical-record reviews verified more than 90% of self-reported reasons for clinic visits or hospitalizations (Kang et al., 2000).

A followup study of the same population (Kang et al., 2009) was conducted in 2005 to obtain survey-based health information from the 15,000 Gulf War–deployed and 15,000 Gulf War–era veterans originally surveyed in 1995. In phase I of the followup, VA and Social Security records through December 2002 were used to identify the 29,607 living participants and mail health questionnaires to them. Phase II consisted of telephone interviews with 2,000 participants who did not respond to the initial mailed questionnaire (nonrespondents) and a sample of 1,000 participants (respondents) who had indicated a clinic visit or hospitalization within the previous 12 months. In all, 6,111 (40%) deployed and 3,859 (27%) nondeployed veterans participated in both phases I and II, but the overall response rate was low (only 34%). However, there were no differences in deployment status between respondents and nonrespondents. The administered questionnaire was a modified version of the 1995 questionnaire and included the Patient Health Questionnaire, the 12-Item Short Form Health Survey (SF-12), and other items used to assess general health status. Unexplained multisymptom illness, in this study, was defined as having several symptoms that persisted for 6 months or longer and were not adequately explained by other diagnoses. Those symptoms included fatigue; muscle or joint pain; headache; memory, digestive, respiratory, or skin problems; or any other unexplained symptoms. Unexplained multisymptom illness was identified in 36.5% of the deployed and 11.7% of the era veterans, for a risk ratio of 3.05 (95% confidence interval [CI] 2.77–3.36), after adjustment for age, sex, race, body mass index, current cigarette smoking, rank, branch of service, and unit component (active duty, National Guard, or reserve). Multisymptom

TABLE 3.2 Results of Department of Veterans Affairs Study[a]

Most Common Self-Reported Symptoms	Prevalence in Gulf War Veterans (%)	Prevalence in Non–Gulf War Veterans (%)
Runny nose	56	43
Headache	54	37
Unrefreshing sleep	47	24
Anxiety	45	28
Joint pain	45	27
Back pain	44	30
Fatigue	38	15
Ringing in ears	37	23
Heartburn	37	25
Difficulty in sleeping	37	21
Depression	36	22
Difficulty in concentrating	35	13
5 Most Common Self-Reported Chronic Medical Conditions		
Sinusitis	38.6	28.1
Gastritis	25.2	11.7
Dermatitis	25.1	12.0
Arthritis	22.5	16.7
Frequent diarrhea	21.2	5.9

[a]Subjects were asked whether symptoms were recurring or persistent during previous year. Differences in prevalence are all statistically significant ($p < 0.05$).

SOURCE: Kang et al., 2000. Adapted with permission from Lippincott Williams and Wilkins/Wolters Kluwer Health: *Journal of Occupational and Environmental Medicine* (2000).

illness was the most widely reported medical condition in Gulf War veterans except for arthritis. Gulf War veterans also had higher rates of functional impairment, of limitations of activities, of at least one clinic or doctor visit, and of hospitalization.

The Iowa Study

The Iowa study was a cross-sectional survey of a sample of 4,886 military personnel who listed Iowa as their home of record at the time of enlistment (Iowa Persian Gulf Study Group, 1997). The study examined the health of military personnel in all branches of service who were still serving or had left service. The sample was randomly selected from the 28,968 military personnel who listed Iowa as their home of record. Of the study subjects who were contacted, 3,695 (90.7%) completed a telephone interview in 1995–1996. Study subjects were divided into four groups: Gulf War–deployed regular military, Gulf War–deployed National Guard or reserve, non–Gulf War–deployed regular military, and non–Gulf War–deployed National Guard or reserve. Trained examiners used standardized questions, instruments, and scales in interviewing the subjects.[2] The study found that Gulf War veterans had significantly higher prevalences of symptoms of depression (17.0% vs 10.9%, $p < 0.001$), posttraumatic stress disorder (PTSD; 1.9% vs 0.8%, $p = 0.007$), chronic fatigue (1.3% vs 0.3%, $p < 0.001$), cognitive dysfunction (18.7% vs 7.6%, $p < 0.001$), bronchitis (3.7% vs 2.7%, $p < 0.001$), asthma (7.2% vs 4.1%, $p = 0.004$), fibromyalgia (19.2% vs 9.6%, $p < 0.001$), alcohol abuse (17.2% vs 4.1%, $p = 0.02$), and anxiety (4.0% vs 1.8%, $p < 0.001$). Gulf War veterans scored significantly lower on all eight subscales for physical and mental health on the 36-item Short Form Health Survey (SF-36); this indicated lower quality of life than that of nondeployed personnel. The subscales for bodily pain, general health, and vitality showed the greatest differences between deployed and nondeployed veterans (Iowa Persian Gulf Study Group, 1997). In short, this large, well-controlled study demonstrated that some sets of symptoms were more frequent in Gulf War veterans than in nondeployed military controls.

Oregon and Washington Veteran Studies

Veterans from Oregon and Washington were studied in a series of analyses by investigators of the Portland Environmental Hazards Research Center (McCauley et al., 1999). A mailed questionnaire, to assess general health through symptom self-reports, was sent to a random sample of 2,343 of the total of 8,603 Gulf War veterans who listed Oregon or Washington as their home state of record at the time of deployment. The study did not include a nondeployed comparison group. The response rate was 48.4%. The study found high rates (21–60%) of self-reported symptoms, including cognitive–psychologic symptoms, unexplained fatigue, musculoskeletal pain, gastrointestinal complaints, and rashes. The 225 veterans who participated in the clinical examinations displayed differences between the symptoms that they reported on questionnaires and the symptoms that they reported at clinical examination. The difference might suggest high rates of outcome misclassification based on either the questionnaire or the examination.

Kansas Veteran Study

Kansas established the Kansas Persian Gulf War Veterans Health Initiative to determine the patterns of veterans' health problems. Using lists of eligible veterans from DOD, Steele (2000) conducted a population-based survey of veterans who listed Kansas as their home state of record. A stratified random sample of 3,138 was selected, of whom 2,396 were located with in-state contact information. The survey, mailed out in 1998, asked about 16 specific medical or psychiatric conditions, 37 symptoms, service branch, locations during the Gulf War (including whether the veterans were notified about the Khamisiyah demolitions; see Chapter 2), and vaccinations. Kansas Gulf War veterans reported greater prevalences of 10 physician-diagnosed conditions than Kansas nondeployed veterans: skin conditions, stomach or intestinal conditions, depression, arthritis, migraine headaches, chronic fatigue syndrome (CFS), bronchitis, PTSD, asthma, and thyroid conditions. The investigators used their own definition of Gulf War illness, which was similar to that used by the Centers for Disease Control and Prevention (CDC) (Fukuda et al., 1998) and which required having at least one moderately severe or two or more

[2]Sources of questions included the National Health Interview Survey, the Behavioral Risk Factor Surveillance Survey, the National Medical Expenditures Survey, the Primary Care Evaluation of Mental Disorders, the Brief Symptom Inventory, the CAGE questionnaire (for alcoholism), the PTSD (Posttraumatic Stress Disorder) Checklist—Military, the Centers for Disease Control and Prevention Chronic Fatigue Syndrome Questionnaire, the Chalder Fatigue Scale, the American Thoracic Society questionnaire, and the Sickness Impact Profile.

chronic symptoms in at least three of six domains: fatigue and sleep problems; pain symptoms; neurologic, cognitive, and mood symptoms; gastrointestinal symptoms; respiratory symptoms; and skin symptoms. The symptoms had to persist or recur in the year before the study interview and had to have been a problem for the study participants in 1990 or later. Using their case definition, the researchers found that 34.2% of Gulf War veterans and 8.3% of nondeployed veterans met criteria for Gulf War illness (odds ratio [OR] = 4.68, 95% CI 3.25–6.75). On the basis of the CDC case criteria, the study found that 47.2% of Gulf War veterans and 19.8% of nondeployed veterans had chonic multisymptom illness (OR = 3.26, 95% CI 2.48–4.28). The prevalence of Kansas-defined Gulf War illness was lowest in Gulf War veterans who served on ships and highest in those who served in Iraq or Kuwait.

Canadian Veteran Study

A 1997 survey mailed to the entire cohort of Canadian Gulf War veterans found high prevalences of several chronic conditions (Goss Gilroy Inc., 1998).[3] Some 3,113 respondents from Canada who had been deployed to the Gulf War were compared with 3,439 respondents who had been deployed elsewhere during the same period. The Gulf War veterans who responded reported symptoms of cognitive dysfunction, multiple chemical sensitivity (MCS), major depression, PTSD, chronic dysphoria, anxiety, and respiratory diseases at higher rates than the controls. The greatest differences between Gulf War–deployed forces and those deployed elsewhwere were in symptoms of cognitive dysfunction, MCS, and major depression. Symptoms of cognitive dysfunction had the highest overall prevalence: in 34–40% of Gulf War veterans and 10–15% of veterans deployed elsewhere. Gulf War veterans also reported significantly more visits to health care practitioners, greater dissatisfaction with their health status, and greater health-related reductions in recent activity.

United Kingdom Veteran Studies

The United Kingdom sent 53,000 personnel to the Gulf War. Two teams of researchers each studied a separate, nonoverlapping, stratified random sample of those Gulf War veterans. The first team was from the University of London (Guy's, King's, and St. Thomas's Medical Schools), the second team from the University of Manchester. A third team of researchers from the London School of Hygiene and Tropical Medicine surveyed the entire cohort of 53,000 veterans for a focused study of birth defects and other reproductive outcomes.

University of London Veteran Studies

Unwin et al. (1999) at the University of London investigated the health of UK servicemen in a population-based study. The study used a random sample of the entire UK contingent deployed to the Gulf War and two comparison groups. One of the comparison groups (n = 2,620) was deployed to the conflict in Bosnia; this is the only study that used a comparison population that had combat experience during the time of the Gulf War. The second comparison group of era veterans (n = 2,614) was deployed to noncombat locations outside the United Kingdom in the same period. As opposed to what was done in some studies, the nondeployed control group was recruited from among the subset of nondeployed service members who were

---

[3]In January 1997, Goss Gilroy Inc. was contracted by the Canadian Department of National Defence to carry out an epidemiologic survey of Canadians who served in the Gulf War to establish the overall health status of Gulf War personnel.

fit for combat duty, and this avoided selection bias related to the healthy-warrior effect. A mailed questionnaire queried symptoms (50 items), medical disorders (39 items), exposure history (29 items), and functional capacity. The authors compared ORs for each symptom after controlling for potential confounding factors (including sociodemographic and lifestyle factors), using logistic regression analysis. Only results on male veterans were analyzed, because female veterans' roles and symptoms were distinct enough to warrant separate consideration. Responses to the questionnaire were received from 70% of the 53,462 Gulf War–deployed, 61.9% of the 39,217 in the Bosnia cohort, and 62.9% of the 250,000 era cohort members. Bosnia-deployed veterans were more likely to be in service, unmarried, younger, and drank more alcohol than Gulf War–deployed veterans. The era veterans were similar to Gulf War–deployed veterans but included more non-smokers.

The Gulf War–deployed veterans (n = 2,961) reported higher prevalences of symptoms and diminished functioning than did either comparison group. Gulf War veterans were 2–3 times more likely than comparison subjects to have met symptom-based criteria for chronic fatigue, posttraumatic stress reaction, and CDC-defined chronic multisymptom illness (CMI; Fukuda et al., 1998). More specifically, 25.3% of Gulf War veterans met CDC case criteria for CMI compared with 11.8% of Bosnia and 12.2% of Gulf War–era veterans. The most frequently reported symptoms were feeling unrefreshed after sleep, irritability or outbursts of anger, headache, fatigue, sleeping difficulties, forgetfulness, joint stiffness, loss of concentration, flatulence or burping, pain without swelling, and redness in several joints. Gulf War veterans were 2–3 times more likely to report those symptoms, but results were not statistically significant. On the SF-36, Gulf War veterans reported significantly worse health perception but not worse physical functioning. It should be noted that the members of the Bosnia cohort, who also had been deployed to a combat setting, reported fewer symptoms than the Gulf War cohort, and this suggests that combat deployment itself does not necessarily account for higher symptom reporting (Unwin et al., 1999).

In a followup study, a postal survey was sent 11 years after the war to a random sample of 3,305 participants (1,472 Gulf War–deployed, 909 Bosnia-deployed, and 924 era veterans) from the total who completed the first study described above. The response rates were as follows: 74.0% Gulf War–deployed, 70.2% Bosnia-deployed, and 69.7% era veterans. Respondents completed the Chalder fatigue scale, the General Health Questionnaire (GHQ), SF-36, and the count of physical symptoms (Hotopf et al., 2003). Compared with the first survey (time 1), respondents reported a modest reduction in fatigue, modest reduction in psychologic distress on the GHQ, and slight worsening on SF-36. Compared with the two groups of non–Gulf War–deployed veterans surveyed at time 2, deployed veterans performed worse on all measures. Deployed veterans reported a mean of 10.7 symptoms vs 7.9 and 6.4 in the two non–Gulf War–deployed veteran groups. They had no higher incidence of new illnesses.

University of Manchester Veteran Study

The University of Manchester study used a random sample of UK veterans 7 years after the Gulf War (Cherry et al., 2001). The cohort was deliberately separate from that studied by Unwin et al. (1999). The 9,505 eligible deployed veterans were divided into two groups—4,755 in the main cohort and 4,750 in a validation cohort to permit replication of analysis and to assess consistency. The control population of 4,749 consisted of nondeployed veterans who were in good general health. Veterans were sent a questionnaire about the extent to which they were burdened by 95 symptoms in the previous month. By asking them to mark their answers on a visual analogue scale, investigators sought to determine the degree of symptom severity. Investigators also sought to determine areas of peripheral neuropathy by asking veterans to shade on two pictures of mannequins the body areas where they were experiencing pain or numbness and tingling. Deployed veterans reported greater severity of almost all 95 symptoms. The overall mean severity scores of the two Gulf War cohorts were similar and significantly greater than the score of the non–Gulf War cohort. Deployed veterans' severity scores for 14 symptoms—including memory, concentration, and mood problems—were at least twice those of the nondeployed veterans. Numbness and tingling were reported by about 13% of deployed and about 7% of nondeployed. Widespread pain was also reported more frequently (12.2% vs 6.5%).

London School of Hygiene and Tropical Medicine Veteran Study

The third British study was a large mail survey conducted by researchers at the London School of Hygiene and Tropical Medicine (Maconochie et al., 2003; Simmons et al., 2004). It was designed largely to assess reproductive outcomes in Gulf War veterans, but it contained open-ended questions about their general health. The exposed cohort consisted of all UK Gulf War veterans, and the unexposed cohort consisted of a random sample of nondeployed UK military personnel from the same period. Although the number of surveys returned in the study was large (25,084 by Gulf War veterans and 19,003 by non–Gulf War veterans), the participation rates were low (47.3% and 37.5% of male and female Gulf War veterans, respectively, and 57.3% and 45.6% of male and female nondeployed veterans, respectively). Simmons et al. (2004) reported that 61% of responding Gulf War veterans and 37% of responding nondeployed veterans reported at least one new medical symptom or disease since 1990. Some 85% of symptoms and diseases were reported more frequently by Gulf War veterans. The strongest associations were for mood swings (OR = 20.9, 95% CI 16.2–27.0), memory loss or lack of concentration (OR = 19.6, 95% CI 15.5–24.8), night sweats (OR = 9.9, 95% CI 6.5–15.2), general fatigue (OR = 9.6, 95% CI 8.3–11.1), and sexual dysfunction (OR = 4.6, 95% CI 3.2–6.6). Adjustments were made for age, service, rank, serving status, alcohol consumption, and smoking. Veterans' belief that they had "Gulf War syndrome" was associated with the greater reporting of symptoms or disease, but only 6% of Gulf War veterans believed that they had the syndrome.

Danish Peacekeeper Studies

Military personnel from Denmark were involved in peacekeeping or humanitarian missions that occurred predominantly after the Gulf War ceasefire but were in the same areas as other coalition forces that served in Gulf War combat (Ishøy et al., 1999). A total of 821 Danes, deployed from August 1990 to December 1997, were eligible for inclusion in this population-based cohort, and 686 (83.6%) agreed to participate in the study. The deployed veterans were matched by age, sex, and profession to 400 members of the Danish armed forces who were not deployed to the Gulf War; 231 (57.8%) agreed to participate. Participants completed a detailed questionnaire, including 22 neuropsychologic symptoms, and then received detailed clinical health and laboratory examinations (height, weight, blood pressure, a battery of urinary and blood work, and a battery of neuropsychologic tests) and participated in physician interviews about their medical history and symptoms. The examinations were conducted in 1997–1998.

The results showed that Danish peacekeepers were significantly more likely to have a wide variety of symptoms (with onset during or after August 2, 1990), including headache, blurry vision, numbness or tingling of hands or feet, balance difficulties, depression and concentration problems, fatigue, sleep difficulty, nightmares, nervousness and agitation, and difficulty in pronouncing words. Analyses did not adjust for potential confounders. All together, Gulf War veterans reported higher prevalences of 17 of 22 neuropsychologic symptoms, 8 of 14 gastrointestinal symptoms, and 8 of 19 skin symptoms. Rates of symptoms that appeared before August 2, 1990, were no different among groups. Only minor differences were found among the groups in hematologic measures (Ishøy et al., 1999). The authors concluded that because Danish peacekeepers' symptoms were consistent with American Gulf War veterans' symptoms, results indicate the existence of some common risk factors that are independent of combat.

Australian Veteran Studies

Investigators at Monash University conducted a cohort study of Australian service personnel who had (1,456) or had not (1,588) been deployed to the gulf as part of the multinational force (Kelsall et al., 2004). Participation rates were 80.5% and 56.8%, respectively. In the Australian contingent sent to the Gulf War, members of the Navy were heavily overrepresented (86.5%). Participants completed mailed questionnaires: a physical and mental health screening questionnaire (SF-12), a test for nonpsychotic psychologic illness (GHQ-12), a PTSD checklist (PCL-S), and a questionnaire about military service and exposures.

Kelsall et al. (2004) stated that participants in the deployed cohort reported higher prevalences of all 63 symptoms (all but seven were statistically significant) and reported more severe symptoms. The symptoms that had the highest prevalences were feeling unrefreshed after sleep (adjusted OR = 1.6, 95% CI 1.3–1.8), fatigue (adjusted OR = 1.6, 95% CI 1.3–1.8), headache (adjusted OR = 1.3, 95% CI 1.1–1.6), sleeping difficulties (adjusted OR = 1.6, 95% CI 1.4–1.9), and irritability and outbursts of anger (adjusted OR = 1.6, 95% CI 1.4–1.8).

French Military Study

Salamon et al. (2006) surveyed all French troops who were deployed to the Gulf War. The study was able to survey 5,666 of 20,261 French veterans (28% response rate) and perform clinical examinations on 1,008. On the basis of a health questionnaire administered from 2002 to 2004, the study found that signs, symptoms, and ill-defined (SSID) conditions were self-reported by 10.9% of Gulf War veterans. Among all participants, the symptoms reported most often were headache (82.9%), sleeping difficulties (70.9%), irritability (68.8%), backache (62.9%), and memory difficulties (56.0%).

MILITARY UNIT–BASED STUDIES

Hawaii and Pennsylvania Active-Duty and Reserve Study

One of the first epidemiologic studies of US Gulf War veterans examined the psychologic and physical health of active-duty and reserve Army, Navy, Air Force, and Marine Corps personnel from bases in Pennsylvania and Hawaii (Stretch et al., 1995). Questionnaires were mailed to 14,167 potential study participants with questions regarding demographics; physical, psychologic, and psychosocial symptoms; deployment type; and perceived sources of stress before, during, and after combat or deployment. A total of 4,334 veterans returned the questionnaires, for a response rate of 31%. Of those, 715 active-duty personnel and 766 reserves were deployed to the Gulf War, and 1,576 active-duty personnel and 948 reserves were not deployed; the remainder deployed to other locations. Significantly more deployed personnel reported 20 of 23 queried symptoms than nondeployed personnel. For 12 symptoms, deployed personnel were more than twice as likely as nondeployed personnel to report head colds, sinus trouble, sore throat, difficulty swallowing, headaches, back problems, stomach upset, muscle aches, aching joints, cough, chills or fever, and "other problems." Adjusted ORs for those symptoms ranged from 2.14 to 3.76 (all $p < 0.001$)—adjustments were made for age, rank, education, marital status, and branch of military.

Ft. Devens and New Orleans Cohort Studies

The symptom experience of two deployed cohorts of Gulf War veterans was studied by Boston-based researchers (Proctor et al., 1998; Wolfe et al., 1998). The first, an Army cohort based in Ft. Devens, Massachusetts, was surveyed longitudinally at three times (1991, 1993–1994, and 1997). The second Gulf War deployed cohort was from New Orleans. The study's 252 subjects were the result of a stratified random sample of 2,949 troops from Ft. Devens and 928 from New Orleans; both groups consisted of active-duty, reserve, and National Guard troops. A third unit consisted of 48 members of an air-ambulance company of National Guard from Maine that had been deployed to Germany for handling wounded personnel evacuated from the gulf.

In comparison with veterans deployed to Germany during the Gulf War era, random samples of both Gulf War cohorts had higher prevalences of 51 of 52 items on a health-symptom checklist (Proctor et al., 1998). The greatest differences in prevalence of reported symptoms were of dermatologic symptoms (such as rash, eczema, and skin allergies), neuropsychologic symptoms (such as difficulty in concentrating and difficulty in learning new material), and gastrointestinal symptoms (such as stomach cramps and excessive gas). With a separate checklist, researchers found a higher prevalence of PTSD, according to the Clinician-Administered PTSD Scale (5% Ft. Devens, 7% New Orleans, and 0% Germany). The Ft. Devens group reported significantly higher rates of 35 of the 52 symptoms than the unit in Germany. The New Orleans group reported significantly higher prevalences of 24 of the 52. Among the musculoskeletal symptoms reported more frequently by the Ft. Devens deployed veterans were joint pains (OR = 2.6) and neck aches or stiffness (OR = 2.7), and among the neurologic symptoms with greater prevalences in both cohorts of deployed veterans was headache (OR = 4.2); all were statistically significant. About 30% of the Gulf War veterans and 11% of the comparison group reported an inability to fall asleep (OR 3.4–3.6, $p \leq 0.05$).

In a subanalysis of 2,119 veterans in the Ft. Devens cohort conducted in 1993, Wolfe et al. (1998) reported on symptoms on a 20-item symptom checklist. They found that the most frequent symptoms were general aches and pains, being overly tired/lack of energy, headaches, trouble sleeping, nervous or tense, depressed mood, and difficulty concentrating. Some 30% of the sample reported that their physical health had become either "worse" or "much worse" since their return.

Seabee Reserve Battalion Studies

Numerous studies of the Seabees called to active duty for the Gulf War have been conducted. Haley et al. (1997) studied members of the Twenty-Fourth Reserve Naval Construction Battalion who lived in five southern states and were called to active duty. The unit was a mobile construction battalion for other branches of the military. More than half the battalion's members had left the military by the time of the study and so were not included in the study cohort. Participants were recruited among those whose addresses were available and from veterans' meetings. Of the 249 participants, 175 (70%) reported having had serious health problems since returning from the Gulf War. A telephone survey of a random sample of nonparticipants found that although they were demographically similar to participants, fewer (43%) reported having had serious health problems since the war. Some 11% of participants and 3% of nonparticipants were unemployed. Of the 606 men in the battalion, 41.1% participated; there was no nondeployed group for comparison. The study was the first to cluster symptoms into new syndromes by applying factor-analysis techniques (discussed in Chapter 4).

In the first of a series of studies by Gray et al. (1999), investigators surveyed active-duty Seabees who remained on active duty for at least 3 years after the Gulf War. The Seabees were in 14 Seabee commands at two locations (Port Hueneme, California, and Gulfport, Mississippi). Those who were deployed to the Gulf War were in mobile construction battalions serving in the same tasks and at the same sites as the reserve Seabee battalion studied by Haley and collaborators. During the Gulf War, Seabees built airports, supply points, and roads. Gray et al. (1999) excluded Gulf War veterans who were no longer active at the time of the study in 1994–1995.

Gray et al. (1999) enrolled 1,497 study subjects: 527 Gulf War–deployed veterans and 970 nondeployed veterans. Study subjects filled out symptom and exposure questionnaires and answered additional questions that screened for PTSD, CFS, and various psychologic symptom domains; blood and handgrip strength were also tested. The study had a 53% participation rate. Findings indicated that 55.8% of Gulf War–deployed and 31.7% of nondeployed era veterans reported prolonged symptoms (lasting for 1 month or longer) that occurred after the war; the prevalences of 35 of 41 symptoms were significantly higher in the deployed than in the nondeployed. The groups had similar pulmonary function and reactant assays (C-reactive protein, transferrin, and haptoglobin). Gulf War veterans had higher adjusted serum ferritin measurements, but results were within the normal range. Handgrip strength was lower in Gulf War veterans on the average, and they were more likely to have PTSD (15% vs 9%).

Beginning in May 1997, Gray et al. (2002) mailed a questionnaire to all 18,945 regular and reserve naval personnel who served on active-duty Seabee command during the Gulf War period. The questionnaire collected information regarding medical history, current health status, symptoms and medical problems, and environmental exposures. Of the 17,559 participants located, 11,868 completed and returned the questionnaire: 3,831 Gulf War–deployed, 4,933 deployed elsewhere, and 3,104 nondeployed. Compared with the two control groups, the deployed were more likely to report having more symptoms; the greatest differences were evident in MCS, nightmares or flashbacks, rash or skin ulcer, general muscle weakness, and unusual irritability. Gulf War–deployed Seabees were significantly more likely to report having more of all 33 self-reported medical problems than personnel in the other two groups on the basis of logistic regression analyses that controlled for age, sex, race or ethnicity, and duty status. Gulf War–deployed Seabees were also significantly more likely to report suffering from a wide variety of physician-diagnosed disorders than those nondeployed or deployed elsewhere, including CFS, PTSD, MCS, and irritable bowel syndrome (IBS). Gulf War–deployed Seabees also reported more depression, cognitive failure, digestive diseases, lost work days, and were more likely to report being in fair or poor health than the other two groups. Of the Gulf War–

deployed Seabees, 22% met criteria for Gulf War illness, which the authors defined as having any of five conditions: a self-reported physician diagnosis of CFS, PTSD, MCS, or IBS or self-reporting of 12 or more other medical problems or symptoms. The percentage of members of the control groups meeting the case definition was not reported.

Pennsylvania Air National Guard Study

In response to requests from DOD, VA, and Pennsylvania, a team of investigators from CDC conducted a study to assess health status and prevalence and causes of unexplained illness in Gulf War–deployed personnel (Fukuda et al., 1998). The index unit consisted of 667 members of active-duty Air National Guard members. Three demographically similar Air Force units were used as comparison groups: Unit A consisted of 538 personnel from the Pennsylvania Air National Guard who had a mission different from that of the index unit, Unit B consisted of 838 members of a US Air Force Reserve unit, and Unit C consisted of 1,680 active-duty Air Force personnel from Florida who had a mission similar to that of the index unit. Questionnaires regarding military characteristics, demographics, health status, and 35 specific symptoms previously identified to be of concern were distributed and completed by 3,675 participants (taken together these units included 1,155 Gulf War veterans and 2,520 nondeployed veterans). Response rates were as follows: index unit, 62%; Unit A, 35%; Unit B, 73%; and Unit C, 70%. To assess symptom prevalence, the investigators combined the four units and compared questionnaire responses of deployed and nondeployed. Of 3,723 participants surveyed, those deployed to the Gulf War experienced higher prevalences of chronic symptoms than nondeployed veterans (33 of 35 symptoms of more than 6-month duration were reported to be more prevalent).

Air Force Women's Study

Only one study was devoted to the effects of deployment on symptoms in women. Pierce (1997) surveyed by mail questionnaire 525 US Air Force women who had and had not deployed to the Gulf War. The survey was conducted in 1993 (time 1) and again in 1995 (time 2). Response rates were 82% at time 1 and 92% at time 2. The sampling was random with oversampling of those deployed to the theater of operations and of reserve and National Guard components to achieve a representative study sample. Analyses were adjusted for age. At time 1, the study found that deployed veterans reported rash, cough, depression, unintentional weight loss, insomnia, and memory problems more frequently than nondeployed veterans; differences were not statistically significant, but differences were apparent when data were stratified by duration of deployment to the Gulf. At time 2, the most commonly reported symptoms were rash, cough, memory problems, and sex-specific problems, such as breast lumps or cysts and abnormal pap smears. The pattern of symptom reporting was similar to that by men and women in other Gulf War studies (Unwin et al., 2002).

REGISTRY STUDIES

Several registries have been formed to track and collect information to assist in the investigation of health concerns related to service in the Gulf War. The committee reviewed the registry studies with caution. Registry participants cannot be considered representative of all Gulf War veterans in that they are self-selected subjects, many of whom have joined the registries because they believe that they have symptoms related to Gulf War illness; they were not randomly selected from all Gulf War military personnel, and there is not a nondeployed control group.

In 1992, VA developed and implemented the Persian Gulf Registry. Its original purposes were to ease returning veterans into the VA health care system, to create a registry containing medical and other data on Persian Gulf veterans that would assist in addressing questions about possible future effects of exposure to air pollutants and other environmental agents, and to serve as a basis of future medical surveillance. Exposures, particularly those associated with the oil-well fires, were included as part of the registrants' history. As time passed, it became apparent that a number of exposures and a host of symptoms being reported needed further investigation.

DOD also developed and implemented a Persian Gulf clinical program to diagnose and treat conditions in active-duty military personnel who had medical complaints that they attributed to service in the Gulf War. DOD and VA collaborated and used experts to develop clinical protocols; by 1994, they had implemented similar and parallel clinical evaluation programs. In light of continuing concern about the potential health consequences of service in the Persian Gulf, DOD and VA revised their clinical programs to improve diagnosis of veterans' health complaints. DOD instituted the Comprehensive Clinical Evaluation Program (CCEP), and VA instituted the Persian Gulf Registry and Uniform Case Assessment Protocol (UCAP). Both programs included a medical history, physical examinations, laboratory tests, and specialty consultation as needed. By early 1994, more than 20,000 veterans had been examined as part of VA's Persian Gulf Registry program (IOM, 1998, 1997).

Department of Defense Registry Studies

Four investigations have used the CCEP to identify cohorts for study. A study of the first 20,000 cases seen in the first phase of the CCEP was conducted by Joseph et al. (1997). Findings indicate that 17.8% of Gulf War veterans in the registry had SSID, the most common of which were fatigue, headache, memory problems, and sleep disturbances. In the Gulf War veterans who indicated a date of onset, symptoms were reported to have begun more than 6 months after return from the Gulf War. Gulf War veterans who had SSID did not have any characteristic signs of disease or consistent laboratory abnormalities.

Kroenke et al. (1998) reported on findings from a provider-administered symptom questionnaire on 18,495 Gulf War veterans from the CCEP. The most common symptoms found were joint pain, fatigue, headache, memory and concentration difficulties, sleep disturbance, and rash. The study tracked timing of onset of symptoms relative to the war. Symptom onset was found to be delayed: 66% of symptoms did not appear until after the war, and 40% more than 1 year after the war. According to the authors, there was no association between individual symptoms, types of combat experience, self-reported exposures, or patient demographics. Increased symptom counts were associated with loss of work, the number of self-reported exposures, the number of types of combat experience, and particular *International Classification of Diseases, Ninth Revision* (ICD-9) diagnostic categories (such as psychologic disorders).

Roy et al. (1998) reported on 21,579 Walter Reed Army Medical Center patients who had participated in the CCEP and were referred for additional evaluation. Physicians at Walter Reed conducted a series of evaluations, including a patient health questionnaire, medical history, laboratory studies, and physical examination. The investigators reported that 17.2% of the CCEP participants had a primary diagnosis of SSID, whereas 41.8% had SSID as a primary or secondary diagnosis. The most common symptoms were fatigue, headache, and memory loss. The authors concluded that an analysis of the SSID diagnoses in the large series of Gulf War veterans did not identify a new or unusual syndrome.

Erickson et al. (1998) described musculoskeletal complaints in participants in the CCEP. Of the 1,250 evaluated, 18% were referred to a rheumatologist at the Fitzsimmons Army Medical Center for evaluation of musculoskeletal complaints from March 1994 to March 1995. The most common symptoms reported to rheumatologists were polyarthralgia (pain in more than three joints with or without swelling or widespread pain), knee pain, back pain, myalgia, ankle pain, and hand or wrist pain. Extensive laboratory testing was not specific enough for any diagnosis to explain symptoms.

Department of Veterans Affairs Registry Studies

One of the VA sites, in south Texas, referred 145 potential rheumatologic cases to a nearby clinic (Escalante and Fischbach, 1998). Rheumatologists at the clinic administered a health questionnaire, elicited pain symptoms, and administered the SF-36 for health-related quality of life. Almost all the patients had pain, which was widely distributed and spared no body part. Widespread pain was reported in 65.1% of Gulf War veterans. The most frequent painful areas were knees (in 65%), low back (more than 60%), shoulders (50%), and hands and wrists (35%). The average values on the SF-36 were below the 25th percentile of published national norms. Pain and nonarticular rheumatic symptoms explained most of the diminished health-related quality of life.

Hallman et al. (2003) conducted a health survey in 1995 of 1,161 participating Gulf War veterans who represented a random sample of a VA registry that covered seven states. Of 48 reported symptoms, participants endorsed an average of 9.9 mild symptoms, 9.5 moderate symptoms, and 6.1 severe symptoms. The average total number of symptoms was 25.5.

A 5-year followup of the VA registry members originally surveyed by Hallman et al. (2003) was conducted by Ozakinci et al. (2006). A mail survey was sent to 390 Gulf War veterans who were later interviewed by telephone in 2000 (time 2). Compared with time 1 (1995), there was no significant change in number of symptoms reported or their severity. Subjects who were more symptomatic at time 1 showed some improvement at time 2 but remained much more highly symptomatic than those who had less severe initial symptoms. Adjustments were made for sex, rank, race, marital status, education, branch, and duty.

United Kingdom Registry Study

The health status of 3,000 consecutive registrants in the Gulf Veterans Medical Assessment Programme (GVMAP) was reported by several researchers (Coker et al., 1999; Lee et al., 2001, 2002). The GVMAP provides British Gulf War veterans, who are referred to the program by their regular clinicians, with free specialized health assessments. Some 75% of the registrants were considered well (without organic or psychiatric conditions or able to function normally both physically and mentally): 10% (303) had no conditions or symptoms, 21% (619) complained of symptoms, and 44% had diagnoses of incidental organic or psychiatric illnesses. Among all registrants, the most commonly reported symptoms were affective symptoms (mood, emotions, or feelings), joint and muscle aches and pains, and fatigue.

SUMMARY

Many Gulf War veterans suffer from an array of health problems and symptoms (for example, fatigue, muscle and joint pain, memory loss, gastrointestinal disorders, and rashes) that are not specific to any disease and are not easily classified with standard diagnostic coding systems. Studies since the mid-1990s have found a higher prevalence of self-reported and clinically verified symptoms in Gulf War veterans than in nondeployed Gulf War–era veterans or other control groups. Australian, Canadian, Danish, United Kingdom, and United States Gulf War veterans report higher rates and greater severity of nearly all symptoms or sets of symptoms than their nondeployed counterparts; that finding was reported consistently in every study reviewed by this committee. However, Gulf War veterans do not all experience the same array of symptoms, and the symptoms reported are also found in the nondeployed. Furthermore, the studies are beset with limitations; there is the likelihood that bias distorts the findings and that the representativeness of many, if not most of the studies, is uncertain.

TABLE 3.1 Studies of Symptoms in Gulf War Veterans

Reference	Design	Population	Outcome Measures	Results	Adjustments	Comments
Department of Veterans Affairs Study						
Kang et al., 2000	Cross-sectional survey, conducted in 1995	Population-based sample of 15,000 troops deployed, 15,000 troops not deployed; National Health Survey of Gulf War–era veterans and their families. Includes any person who served in the US military on active duty, in reserves, or in National Guard irrespective of whether they were still in the service or separated. Enrolled 11,441 GWVs and 9,476 NDVs.	Health questionnaire (48-item symptom inventory), functional impairment, limitations of employment, health care use.	GWVs vs NDVs reported higher rates of functional impairment (27.8% vs 14.2%), limitations of employment (17.2% vs 11.6%), and health care use as assessed by clinic visits (50.8% vs 40.5%) or hospitalizations (7.8% vs 6.4%). GWVs reported more frequently all 48 symptoms on health inventory; most frequently severe were back pain, runny nose, joint pain, headaches being anxious, difficulty in getting to sleep, feeling tired, skin rash, excessive fatigue, and heartburn or indigestion.	Sex, branch of service, unit status	Response rate: 70% total, 75% GWVs, 64% NGWs. Compared survey participants with VA health registry participants (n = 15,891). From Kang et al., 2002: 225 NGVs were actually GWVs. Some misclassification in original sample. Assessed selection bias.

Reference	Design	Population	Outcome Measures	Results	Adjustments	Comments
Kang et al., 2009	Followup cross-sectional medical evaluation and survey, conducted in 2005	Derivative of Kang et al. (2000). Eligible population selected randomly from Kang population. Eligible 6,111 GWVs and 3859 NDVs; enrolled 5,469 GWVs and 3,353 NDVs.	Slightly modified version of questionnaire used by Kang et al. (2000) plus Patient Health Questionnaire, SF-12, Multisystem Illness, CFS-like illness.	GWVs vs NDVs have higher rates of multisymptom illness (36.5% vs 11.7%, adjusted RR = 3.05, 95% CI 2.77–3.36), higher rates of CFS-like illness (9.4 vs 3.4, adjusted RR = 2.38, 95% CI 1.97–2.87), more functional impairment (31.6% vs 16.5%), more limitations on activities (29.0% vs 19.2%), higher rates of at least one clinic or doctor visit (56.2% vs 45.9%, $p < 0.001$), and more hospitalizations (10.5% vs 8.0%, $p < 0.001$).	Age, sex, race, body mass, rank, branch of service, unit component (active duty, National Guard, or reserve)	Response rate 34%; differences between respondents and nonrespondents were nondifferential by deployment status.
Iowa Persian Gulf Study						
Iowa Persian Gulf Study Group, 1997	Cross-sectional study; interviews conducted 1995–1996	Iowa listed as home of record on initial military record, and service in regular military or activated National Guard or reserve some time from August 2, 1990, to July 31, 1991. Eligible 4,886; enrolled 1,896 GWVs and 1,799 NDVs.	Telephone interview using standardized questionnaires, instruments, and scales.	GWVs reported significantly higher prevalence of symptoms of depression (17.0% vs 10.9%, $p < 0.001$), PTSD (1.9% vs 0.8%, $p = 0.007$), chronic fatigue (1.3% vs 0.3%, $p < 0.001$), cognitive dysfunction (18.7% vs 7.6%, $p < 0.001$), and fibromyalgia (19.2% vs 9.6%, $p < 0.001$).	Age, sex, race, branch of military, rank	Response rate 76%. Limited assessment of selection bias. Stratum random sample with proportional allocation—64 strata (GW, type of military, age, sex, race, rank, branch).

Reference	Design	Population	Outcome Measures	Results	Adjustments	Comments
Oregon and Washington Veteran Studies						
McCauley et al., 1999	Case-control study, survey, and clinical examination, conducted in 1995–1998	GWV residents of Oregon and Washington in Operation Desert Shield or Desert Storm. Eligible 1,396 GWVs. Enrolled 158 GWVs with unexplained illness and 67 healthy GWV controls.	Unexplained health symptoms reported on mailed questionnaire and symptoms reported at clinical examination. Symptoms were not attributable to organic condition. Emphasis on disease misclassification in cross-sectional surveys.	Significant differences between symptoms reported on survey questionnaire and those confirmed at clinical examination. Self-reported fatigue was confirmed in 79% of participants, self-reported GI symptoms in 20%, and musculoskeletal pain in 35%.		Randomly selected population, reservists oversampled, all women selected. No nondeployed control group. Response rate 32.5% for clinical examination, 53.2% of cases, and 51.5% of controls. Blinded clinicians reviewed case-control status.
Kansas Veteran Study						
Steele, 2000	Cross-sectional survey, cconducted by telephone in 1998	Kansas residents on active duty August 1990–July 1991, separated or retired from military, or currently serving in reserve component. Eligible 3,138; enrolled 1,548 GWVs and 482 NDVs.	37-item symptom questionnaire.	34.2% GWVs and 8.3% NDVs met Kansas criteria for Gulf War illness (OR = 4.68, 95% CI 3.25–6.75). 47.2% GWVs and 19.8% NDVs met CDC case criteria (OR = 3.26, 95% CI 2.48–4.28). Prevalence of Kansas-defined Gulf War illness lowest in GWVs serving on ships and highest in those in Iraq or Kuwait.	Sex, age, income, education level, rank, service branch, component	92% response rate. No assessment of selection bias.
Canadian Veteran Study						
Goss Gilroy Inc., 1998	Cross-sectional postal survey,	All Canadian Gulf War veterans.	Survey of chronic conditions and	GWVs reported higher prevalence of symptoms of	Income and rank were	Response rate 73% GWVs,

Reference	Design	Population	Outcome Measures	Results	Adjustments	Comments
	conducted in 1997	Enrolled 3,113 GWVs and 3,439 veterans deployed elsewhere.	symptoms.	chronic fatigue (OR = 5.27, 95% CI 3.95–7.03), cognitive dysfunction (OR = 4.36, 95% CI 3.80–5.01), MCS (OR = 4.01, 95% CI 2.43–6.62), major depression (OR = 3.67, 95% CI 3.04–4.44), anxiety (OR = 2.20, 95% CI 1.55–3.12), PTSD (OR = 2.69, 95% CI 1.69–4.26), chronic dysphoria (OR = 2.68, 95% CI 2.13–3.35), fibromyalgia (OR = 1.81, 95% CI 1.55–2.13), and respiratory diseases (OR = 1.35, 95% CI 1.16–1.57) than veterans deployed elsewhere (all $p < 0.05$). 47% of GWV and 74% of controls did not report any health outcome.	important confounders; sex did not affect associations	60% controls. 189 respondents were female. Controls were age- and sex-matched. Also compared with general population using 1990 Ontario Health Survey.
United Kingdom Veteran Studies						
Unwin et al., 1999	Cross-sectional survey, conducted in 1997–1998	Stratified random sample of 53,462 UK military who served in gulf region, excluding special forces, compared with 39,217 personnel who served in Bosnia in 1992–1997 and 250,000 era cohort in military but not	50-item symptom questionnaire, SF-36, GHQ.	25.3% of GWVs, 11.8% Bosnia, and 12.2% era cohort met CDC case criteria. GWVs reported higher rates of all 50 symptoms. Most frequent symptoms were feeling unrefreshed after sleep, irritability or outbursts of anger, headache, fatigue, sleeping difficulties, forgetfulness, joint stiffness, loss of concentration, flatulence or burping, and pain without swelling or redness in several joints. SF-36	Age, smoking, alcohol consumption, marital status, education, rank, employment, civilian or military status	Response rates 70% GWVs, 63% Bosnia cohort, 62% era cohort. Authors note that 800 Bosnian veterans later moved to GWV group. Extensive assessment of selection bias. Stratified by

Reference	Design	Population	Outcome Measures	Results	Adjustments	Comments
		gulf in 1991. Enrolled 2,961 GWVs, 2,620 Bosnia, and 2,614 NDVs.		significantly worse in GWVs' health perception but not physical functioning.		service, sex, age, service status, rank, fitness. Oversampled women.
Hotopf et al., 2003	Cross-sectional survey, conducted in 2000–2001	Followup of Unwin et al. (1999). Selected all women; all male veterans with fatigue score >8; 50% sample of GWVs, with scores 4–8, all 4–8 in Bosnia and era; 1 in 8 sample of veterans with scores <4. Enrolled 1,089 GWVs, 638 Bosnia, and 634 NDVs.	Chalder Fatigue Scale, GHQ, SF-36, count of physical symptoms.	Modest reduction in fatigue since time 1, modest reduction in psychologic distress on GHQ since time 1, slight worsening on SF-36 since time 1. When compared with two groups of nondeployed veterans, SF-36 was worse, GHQ was worse, and fatigue was worse in GWVs, and they had 10.7 total symptoms in vs 7.9 and 6.4 in NDVs. No higher incidence of new illnesses.	Age, sex, rank, marital status	8,196 reported to first survey (Unwin et al., 1999). Response rate 71.6%.
Cherry et al., 2001	Cross-sectional survey by mailed questionnaire conducted 1997–1999	UK military who served in gulf region September 1990–June 1991, excluding special forces, compared with nondeployed military as January 1, 1991. Total eligible	Health questionnaire surveying 95 symptoms (experienced in preceding month) and two mannequins on which to shade areas of pain or numbness and tingling. Personal followup visits. Factor analysis and	On every symptom, score was higher for GWVs. Symptoms on which score was at least twice as high included difficulty in concentrating, poor memory, sudden changes in mood, feeling too weak to complete what you are doing, and feeling incapable of making decisions. In shading on mannequins, GWVs more likely to report symptoms	Age, rank, still serving, marital status, sex	Sample stratified by sex, age, service, rank. Matched with randomly selected sample of NGVs. Three stratified random samples: main GWVs, GWV validation sample,

Reference	Design	Population	Outcome Measures	Results	Adjustments	Comments
		14,254; enrolled 4,076 GWVs, 4,135 GWVs validation sample, 4,749 NGVs.	cluster analysis.	consistent with peripheral neuropathy: 6.0% limited, 8.5% extended in GWVs vs 4.5% limited, 2.3% extended in NGVs. Widespread pain reported in 12.2% GWVs and 6.5% NGVs.		non-GWVs. Assessed selection bias. Relatively high response rate: 85.5%. No overlap with Unwin et al. (1999).
Maconochie et al., 2003; Simmons et al., 2004	Retrospective cohort study of veterans who believed they had GWS; assessed by mailed questionnaire in 1998–2001	All UK armed forces personnel. Enrolled 24,379 GWVs and 18,439 NDVs.	Incidence of self-reported adult ill health.	61% GWVs and 37% NDVs reported at least one new symptom since 1990. 85% of symptoms or diseases queried were higher in GWVs; strongest associations were in mood swings (OR = 20.9, 95% CI 16.2–27.0), memory loss or lack of concentration (OR = 19.6, 95% CI 15.5–24.8), night sweats (OR = 9.9, 95% CI 6.5–15.2), general fatigue (OR = 9.6, 95% CI 8.3–11.1), and sexual dysfunction (OR = 4.6, 95% CI 3.2–6.6).	Age, service, rank, serving status, alcohol consumption, smoking	47% response rate for men. Analyses restricted to men only for statistical power.
Danish Peacekeeper Studies						
Ishoy et al., 1999	Cross-sectional study with questionnaire and medical examinations; health examinations conducted in 1997–1998	Danish Gulf War veterans stationed in gulf August 2, 1990–December 31, 1997, UN peacekeeping force, officers, noncommissioned officers, and	Questionnaire on neuropsychologic, gastrointestinal, and skin symptoms.	Deployed veterans reported higher prevalence ($p < 0.05$) of 17 of 22 neuropsychologic symptoms, 8 of 14 gastrointestinal symptoms, and 8 of 19 skin symptoms. 81% deployed veterans and 71% controls had one or more ICD-10 diagnoses at examination	None	Response rates 83.6% GWVs 57.8% NGVs. Limited assessment of selection bias (most frequent reason for not participating was

Reference	Design	Population	Outcome Measures	Results	Adjustments	Comments
		enlisted privates compared with Danish armed forces who could have been but had not been deployed in gulf. Eligible 821 GWVs and 400 NDVs; enrolled 686 GWVs and 231 NDVs.		($p = 0.002$).		lack of time). Comparison group matched on sex, age, profession; randomly selected at end of 1996.
Australian Veteran Studies						
Kelsall et al., 2004	Cross-sectional mailed questionnaire and comprehensive health assessment, conducted in 2000–2002	All Australian veterans who served in gulf August 2, 1990–September 4, 1991, compared with 26,411 Australian Defense Force personnel in operational units at the time but not deployed. Eligible 4,795; enrolled 1,456 GWVs and 1,588 NGVs.	63-item symptom questionnaire, medical-condition questionnaire, exposure questionnaire, functional impairment, 44-item military service experience regarding war stressors.	GWVs reported higher rates of all 63 symptoms (all but seven were statistically significant) and reported more severe symptoms. Top 5 symptoms were feeling unrefreshed after sleep (adjusted OR = 1.6, 95% CI 1.3–1.8), fatigue (adjusted OR = 1.6, 95% CI 1.3–1.8), headache (adjusted OR = 1.3, 95% CI 1.1–1.6), sleeping difficulties (adjusted OR = 1.6, 95% CI 1.4–1.9), and irritability or outbursts of anger (adjusted OR = 1.6, 95% CI 1.4–1.8).	Service type, rank, age, education, marital status	Assessed selection bias. Used telephone survey–only results. Response rates: 80.5% GWVs, 56.8% NDVs. Comparison group randomly selected and frequency-matched by service type, age, rank. Limited to men only.
French Military Study						
Salamon et al., 2006	Cross-sectional survey and clinical exam, conducted in	5,666 French GWVs. Eligible 20,261; enrolled 5,666.	Health symptoms and medical conditions, medical evaluation.	SSID self-reported by 10.9% of GWVs. Top five symptoms were headache (82.9%), sleeping difficulties (70.9%), irritability		Response rate: 28%. No nondeployed control group.

Reference	Design	Population	Outcome Measures	Results	Adjustments	Comments
	2002–2004			(68.8%), backache (62.9%), and memory difficulties (56.0%).		1,008 GWVs completed the clinical exam.
Hawaii and Pennsylvania Active-Duty and Reserve Study						
Stretch et al., 1995	Cross-sectional survey of service members from Hawaii and Pennsylvania	16,167 active-duty and reserve personnel assigned to all Army, Navy, Air Force and Marine Corps units in Hawaii and Pennsylvania. Enrolled 1,481 GWVs and 2,524 NDVs.	Health questionnaire.	GWVs were significantly more likely than NDVs to report 12 symptoms: head cold, sinus trouble, sore throat, difficulty swallowing, headache, back problems, stomach upset, muscle aches, aching joints, cough, chills/fever, other problems (all $p < 0.001$).	Age, rank, education, marital status, branch of military	Response rate: 31%. No formal assessment of selection bias (speculated on reasons for nonresponses).
Ft. Devens and New Orleans Cohort Studies						
Proctor et al., 1998	Cross-sectional study of 3 cohorts followed longitudinally; dates of enrollment: Ft. Devens 1991, 1992–1993, 1994–1996; New Orleans 1991, 1994–1995; Germany 1995	Stratified random samples of two Gulf War–deployed groups: Ft. Devens and New Orleans compared with nondeployed group (Germany). Ft. Devens: US Army active, reserve, and National Guard veterans; New Orleans: active, reserve, and National Guard US Army, Navy,	52-item symptom questionnaire.	GWVs report higher prevalence of all but one of 52 symptoms. Ft. Devens group reported significantly higher prevalences than Germany group. New Orleans group reported significantly higher prevalences of 24 of 52 symptoms. Among musculoskeletal symptoms reported more frequently by Ft. Devens–deployed veterans were joint pains (OR = 2.6) and neck ache or stiffness (OR = 2.7); among neurologic symptoms with greater prevalences in both cohorts of deployed veterans was headache (OR = 4.2); all	Age, sex, education	Germany group only studied at time 2. 300 completed Ft. Devens questionnaires were analyzed. Response rates: 53% Ft. Devens, 34% New Orleans, 49% Germany. Assessed selection bias. Oversampled women.

Reference	Design	Population	Outcome Measures	Results	Adjustments	Comments
		Marine Corps, and Air Force troops; Germany: Maine National Guard air ambulance unit. Final participation 252 GWVs (Ft. Devens and New Orleans) and 48 NDVs (Germany).		confidence intervals excluded 1.0. About 30% of Gulf War veterans and 11% of Germany group reported inability to fall asleep (OR = 3.4–3.6, 95% CI excludes 1.0).		
Wolfe et al., 1998	Longitudinal study, cross-sectional survey conducted in 1993	Population included Proctor et al. (1998) sample. GWVs from Ft. Devens. Eligible 2,949; enrolled 2,119.	20-item health-symptom checklist.	Most frequent symptoms were general aches and pains, overtiredness or lack of energy, headache, trouble sleeping, nervous or tense, depressed mood, difficulty concentrating; 30% of sample indicated that their physical health had become either "worse" or "much worse" since their return.	Age, educational level, marital status, race	Response rate: 92%. No NDVs.
Seabee Studies						
Haley et al., 1997	Cross-sectional survey, factor-analysis survey conducted individually in supervised, in-person, group sessions in 1995	Active and retired members of 24th Reserve Naval Mobile Construction Battalion, called to active duty in GW, residents of Alabama, Georgia, North Carolina, South Carolina, and Tennessee in	Self-reported exposure to neurotoxic chemical combinations and association with factor analysis–defined syndrome.	Survey results indicated 6 symptom factors (called syndromes by the authors): impaired cognition, confusion–ataxia, arthromyoneuropathy, phobia–apraxia, fever–adenopathy, and weakness–incontinence. They accounted for 71% of observed variance. 63 (25%) veterans had one of the 6 "syndromes," authors noted. 70% had serious health problems		No assessment of selection bias. Small cohort, no control group. Response rate: 41%. Used cumulative factor weights to assign veterans to "syndromes" with 1.5 cutoff.

Reference	Design	Population	Outcome Measures	Results	Adjustments	Comments
		November 1994. Eligible 606; enrolled 249.		since returning from the Gulf War.		
Gray et al., 1999	Cross-sectional survey conducted in 1994	Active-duty Seabees in Navy in 1994 and serving at Port Hueneme, California, or Gulfport, Mississippi. Eligible 1,497; enrolled 527 GWVs and 970 NDVs.	Questionnaire on postwar symptoms; screening for chronic fatigue and PTSD; Hopkins Symptom Checklist for psychologic symptoms. Clinical evaluation: serum collection, handgrip strength, pulmonary-function testing.	55.8% of GWVs and 31.7% of NGVs reported postwar symptoms lasting ≥1 month. GWVs reported significantly ($p < 0.05$) higher prevalences of 35 out of 41 symptoms than NDVs. Both groups had similar clinical evaluations except GWVs had reduced hand grip strength and were more likely to have PTSD (15% vs 9%) than NDVs.		Assessed selection bias. Response rate: varied by unit, 26–71%.
Gray et al., 2002	Cross-sectional survey conducted in 1997–1999	All regular US Navy Seabees. Eligible 18,945; enrolled 3,831 GWVs, 4,933 veterans deployed elsewhere, and 3,104 NDVs.	Health questionnaire, working case definition.	GWVs reported poor general health, higher prevalences of 33 medical problems, and higher prevalences of CFS, PTSD, MCS, and IBS. 22% met criteria for Gulf War illness.	Age, sex, active-duty or reserve status, race or ethnicity, current smoking, current alcohol drinking	Study limited by recall bias. Response rate: 68.6%. Large sample. Assessed selection bias with telephone survey.
Pennsylvania Air National Guard Study						
Fukuda et al., 1998	Cross-sectional survey conducted in 1995	Everyone on base when survey was conducted was eligible. Index population 667 in ANG unit in Lebanon,	Survey of 35 symptoms, in-person interview. Clinical evaluations of index unit only.	GWV vs NDV: mild to moderate cases 39% vs 14%, severe cases 6% vs 0.7%. Veterans who met case definition had significantly diminished functioning and well-being.	Rank, sex, age, smoking status	Response rates: 61.6% index unit, 35.4% Unit A, 73.4% Unit B, 69.8% Unit C. Deployed to Gulf: 47% index unit,

Reference	Design	Population	Outcome Measures	Results	Adjustments	Comments
		Pennsylvania. Three comparison populations: Unit A, 538 in ANG unit from Pennsylvania with different mission; Unit B, 838 in US Air Force Reserve; Unit C, 1,680 active-duty Air Force from Florida with missions similar to those of index.				22% Unit A, 32% Unit B, 28% Unit C. Started as cluster investigation in Lebanon, Pennsylvania. No assessment of selection bias.
Women in the Air Force						
Pierce, 1997	Cross-sectional survey conducted in 1993 (Time 1) and 1995 (Time 2)	Stratified random sample of women in Air Force. Eligible 638; enrolled 525.	Health survey sex-specific health concerns.	At time 1, symptoms more frequent in GWVs vs NDVs were rash, cough, depression, unintentional weight loss, insomnia, and memory problems. At time 2 symptoms more frequent in GWVs vs NDVs were rash, cough, and memory problems. At time 1, no major difference between GWVs and NDVs in sex-specific symptoms. At time 2, most common symptoms in GWVs were lumps or cysts in breasts, abnormal PAP results, headache, and genital herpes.	Age	Response rates: 82% at time 1, 92% at time 2. 88,415 women in Air Force at the time. Sample composition: 47% active duty, 25.5% reserve, 27.4% Guard.

Reference	Design	Population	Outcome Measures	Results	Adjustments	Comments
Registry Studies						
Joseph et al., 1997	Case series conducted in 1994–1996	Veterans seen by DOD for CCEP. Enrolled 20,000 GWVs.	Physical examination, medical and family history.	17.8% of GWVs had diagnoses of SSID, including primarily fatigue, headache, memory problems, and sleep disturbances		Registry study. Self-selected sample, no control group.
Kroenke et al., 1998	Case series conducted in 1994–1996	Veterans seen by DOD for CCEP Registry. Enrolled 18,495 GWVs.	Provider-administered symptom questionnaire.	Most common symptoms were joint pain (50%), fatigue (46.9%), headache (39.7%), memory or concentration difficulties (34%), sleep disturbance (33%), and rash (30.2%). 66% of symptoms did not appear until after Gulf War, and 40% of symptoms had a latency >1 year. Increased symptom counts were associated with loss of work.		Registry study. Self-selected sample, no control group.
Roy et al., 1998	Case series conducted in 1994–1997	Veterans seen by DOD for Comprehensive Clinical Evaluation Program Registry. Enrolled 21,579 GWVs.	Health questionnaire, physical examination, medical history, laboratory studies.	17.2% of veterans had primary diagnosis of SSID. 41.8% had primary or secondary SSID diagnosis. Most common symptoms were fatigue, headache, sleep disturbance, and memory loss.		Registry study. Self-selected sample, no control group.
Escalante and Fischbach, 1998	Case series of rheumatologic referrals	GWVs enrolled in Persian Gulf Registry from South Texas Veterans Health Care System. Enrolled 145.	Symptoms, self-reported pain, and SF-36 for health-related quality of life.	Pain was present in almost all patients and was widely distributed. Widespread pain was reported in 65.1% of GWVs. Most frequent painful areas were knees (65%), low back (>60%), shoulders (50%),	None	Registry study. Self-selected sample, no control group. Dates of examinations not reported. Registry

Reference	Design	Population	Outcome Measures	Results	Adjustments	Comments
				and hands and wrists (35%). Average values on SF-36 were below 25th percentile of published national norms, with pain and nonarticular rheumatic symptoms explaining most of decrease in health-related quality of life.		enrollment began in 1993.
Hallman et al., 2003	Cross-sectional assessment, conducted in 1995	GWVs residents of Delaware, Illinois, New Jersey, New York, North Carolina, Ohio, and Pennsylvania randomly sampled from VA Gulf War Health Registry. Enrolled 1,161.	Mailed survey.	84.5% attributed their medical problems to service in the gulf. Participants endorsed average of 25.5 symptoms: 9.9 mild, 9.5 moderate, and 6.1 severe.		Registry study. Self-selected sample, no control group. Response rate: 60%. Registry contained more than 70,000 veterans at time of study.
Ozakinci et al., 2006	Cross-sectional assessment, 5-year followup of Hallman et al. (2003) conducted in 2000	Derivative of Hallman et al. (2003). Enrolled 390.	Mailed survey and telephone interview.	Compared with time 1, there was no significant change in number of symptoms reported or their severity. Subjects who were more symptomatic in 1995 showed some improvement but remained much more highly symptomatic than those who were less symptomatic.	Sex, rank, race, marital status, education, branch of service, duty	Response rate: 62%.

Reference	Design	Population	Outcome Measures	Results	Adjustments	Comments
Coker et al., 1999; Lee et al., 2002, 2001	Cross-sectional, case series conducted in 1993–2001	First 3,000 British veterans attending GVMAP.	Medical and psychiatric diagnoses (ICD-10) and nonspecific health symptoms.	75% of first 3,000 GVMAP registrants assessed were well and symptom-free; 21% were well with symptoms but no disease. Most common symptom groups reported were affective (45%), joint and muscle aches and pains (39%), and fatigue (38%). Of registrants assessed as unwell, 11% had psychiatric conditions, 5% organic medical conditions, and 9% both.	None	Registry study. Self-selected sample, no control group.

NOTE: ANG = Air National Guard; CCEP = Comprehensive Clinical Evaluation Program; CDC = Centers for Disease Control and Prevention; CFS = chronic fatigue syndrome; CI = confidence interval; CMI = chronic multisymptom illness; DOD = Department of Defense; GHQ = Global Health Questionnaire; GI = gastrointestinal; GVMAP = Gulf Veterans Medical Assessment Programme; GWS = Gulf War syndrome; GWV = Gulf War veteran; IBS = irritable bowel syndrome; ICD-10 = *International Statistical Classification of Diseases and Related Health Problems, 10th Revision*; MCS = multiple chemical sensitivity; NDV = nondeployed veteran; OR = odds ratio; PTSD = posttraumatic stress disorder; RR = relative risk; SSID = signs, symptoms, and ill-defined conditions; VA = Department of Veterans Affairs.

REFERENCES

Bourdette, D. N., L. A. McCauley, A. Barkhuizen, W. Johnston, M. Wynn, S. K. Joos, D. Storzbach, T. Shuell, and D. Sticker. 2001. Symptom factor analysis, clinical findings, and functional status in a population-based case control study of Gulf War unexplained illness. *Journal of Occupational and Environmental Medicine* 43(12):1026-1040.

Cherry, N., F. Creed, A. Silman, G. Dunn, D. Baxter, J. Smedley, S. Taylor, and G. J. Macfarlane. 2001. Health and exposures of United Kingdom Gulf War veterans. Part II: The relation of health to exposure. *Journal of Occupational and Environmental Medicine* 58(5):299-306.

Coker, W. J., B. M. Bhatt, N. F. Blatchley, and J. T. Graham. 1999. Clinical findings for the first 1000 Gulf War veterans in the Ministry of Defence's Medical Assessment Programme. *British Medical Journal* 318(7179):290-294.

Delgado-Rodríguez, M., and J. Llorca. 2004. Bias. *Journal of Epidemiology and Community Health* 58:635-641.

Erickson, A. R., R. J. Enzenauer, V. J. Bray, and S. G. West. 1998. Musculoskeletal complaints in Persian Gulf War veterans. *Journal of Clinical Rheumatology* 4(4):181-185.

Escalante, A., and M. Fischbach. 1998. Musculoskeletal manifestations, pain, and quality of life in Persian Gulf War veterans referred for rheumatologic evaluation. *Journal of Rheumatology* 25(11):2228-2235.

Fukuda, K., R. Nisenbaum, G. Stewart, W. W. Thompson, L. Robin, R. M. Washko, D. L. Noah, D. H. Barrett, B. Randall, B. L. Herwaldt, A. C. Mawle, and W. C. Reeves. 1998. Chronic multisymptom illness affecting Air Force veterans of the Gulf War. *Journal of the American Medical Association* 280(11):981-988.

Goss Gilroy Inc. 1998. *Health study of Canadian Forces Personnel Involved in the 1991 Conflict in the Persian Gulf.* Ottawa, Canada: Goss Gilroy Inc. Department of National Defence.

Gray, G. C., K. S. Kaiser, A. W. Hawksworth, F. W. Hall, and E. Barrett-Connor. 1999. Increased postwar symptoms and psychological morbidity among U.S. Navy Gulf War veterans. *American Journal of Tropical Medicine and Hygiene* 60(5):758-766.

Gray, G. C., R. J. Reed, K. S. Kaiser, T. C. Smith, and V. M. Gastanaga. 2002. Self-reported symptoms and medical conditions among 11,868 Gulf War-era veterans. *American Journal of Epidemiology* 155(11):1033-1044.

Haley, R. W., T. L. Kurt, and J. Hom. 1997. Is there a Gulf War syndrome? Searching for syndromes by factor analysis of symptoms. *Journal of the American Medical Association* 277(3):215-222. [Erratum appears in *Journal of the American Medical Association* 1997; 278(5):388.]

Hallman, W. K., H. M. Kipen, M. Diefenbach, K. Boyd, H. Kang, H. Leventhal, and D. Wartenberg. 2003. Symptom patterns among Gulf War registry veterans. *American Journal of Public Health* 93(4):624-630.

Hotopf, M., and S. Wessely. 2005. Can epidemiology clear the fog of war? Lessons from the 1990–91 Gulf War. *International Journal of Epidemiology* 34(4):791-800.

Hotopf, M., A. S. David, L. Hull, V. Nikalaou, C. Unwin, and S. Wessely. 2003. Gulf War illness: Better, worse, or just the same? A cohort study. *British Medical Journal* 327(7428):1370-1372.

IOM (Institute of Medicine). 1997. *Adequacy of the Comprehensive Clinical Evaluation Program: A Focused Assessment.* Washington, DC: National Academy Press.

IOM. 1998. *Adequacy of the VA Persian Gulf Registry and Uniform Case Assessment Protocol.* Washington, DC: National Academy Press.

IOM. 1999. *Strategies to Protect the Health of Deployed US Forces: Medical Surveillance, Record Keeping, and Risk Reduction.* Washington, DC: National Academy Press.

IOM. 2006. *Gulf War and Health, Volume 4: Health Effects of Serving in the Gulf War*. Washington, DC: The National Academies Press.

IOM. 2010. *Gulf War and Health, Volume 8: Update of Health Effects of Serving in the Gulf War*. Washington, DC: The National Academies Press.

Iowa Persian Gulf Study Group. 1997. Self-reported illness and health status among Gulf War veterans: A population-based study. *Journal of the American Medical Association* 277(3):238-245.

Ishøy, T., P. Suadicani, B. Guldager, M. Appleyard, and F. Gyntelberg. 1999a. Risk factors for gastrointestinal symptoms: The Danish Gulf War study. *Danish Medical Bulletin* 46(5):420-423.

Ishøy, T., P. Suadicani, B. Guldager, M. Appleyard, H. O. Hein, and F. Gyntelberg. 1999b. State of health after deployment in the Persian Gulf. The Danish Gulf War study. *Danish Medical Bulletin* 46(5):416-419.

Joseph, S. C., R. R. Blanck, G. Gackstetter, R. Glaser, K. C. Hyams, S. Kinty, C. Magruder, J. Mazzuchi, F. L. O'Donnell, M. D. Parkinson, R. E. Patterson, and D. H. Trump. 1997. A comprehensive clinical evaluation of 20,000 Persian Gulf War veterans. *Military Medicine* 162(3):149-155.

Kang, H. K., C. M. Mahan, L. Y. Lee, C. A. Magee, and F. M. Murphy. 2000. Illnesses among United States veterans of the Gulf War: A population-based survey of 30,000 veterans. *Journal of Occupational and Environmental Medicine* 42(5):491-501.

Kang, H. K., C. M. Mahan, K. Y. Lee, F. M. Murphy, S. J. Simmens, H. A. Young, and P. H. Levine. 2002. Evidence for a deployment-related Gulf War syndrome by factor analysis. *Archives of Environmental Health* 57(1):61-68.

Kang, H. K., B. Li, C. M. Mahan, S. A. Eisen, and C. C. Engel. 2009. Health of US Veterans of 1991 Gulf War: A follow-up survey in 10 years. *Journal of Occupational and Environmental Medicine* 51(4):401-410.

Kelsall, H. L., M. R. Sim, A. B. Forbes, D. C. Glass, D. P. McKenzie, J. F. Ikin, M. J. Abramson, L. Blizzard, and P. Ittak. 2004. Symptoms and medical conditions in Australian veterans of the 1991 Gulf War: Relation to immunisations and other Gulf War exposures. *Journal of Occupational and Environmental Medicine* 61(12):1006-1013.

Kelsall, H., R. Macdonell, M. Sim, A. Forbes, D. McKenzie, D. Glass, J. Ikin, and P. Ittak. 2005. Neurological status of Australian veterans of the 1991 Gulf War and the effect of medical and chemical exposures. *International Journal of Epidemiology* 34(4):810-819.

Kroenke, K., P. Koslowe, and M. Roy. 1998. Symptoms in 18,495 Persian Gulf War veterans: Latency of onset and lack of association with self-reported exposures. *Journal of Occupational and Environmental Medicine* 40(6):520-528.

Lee, H. A., R. Gabriel, A. J. Bale, P. Bolton, and N. F. Blatchley. 2001. Clinical findings of the second 1000 UK Gulf War veterans who attended the Ministry of Defence's Medical Assessment programme. *Journal of the Royal Army Medical Corps* 147(2):153-160. [Erratum appears in *Journal of the Royal Army Medical Corps* 2001;147(3):260.]

Lee, H. A., R. Gabriel, J. P. G. Bolton, A. J. Bale, and M. Jackson. 2002. Health status and clinical diagnoses of 3000 UK Gulf War veterans. *Royal Society of Medicine (Great Britain). Journal of the Royal Society of Medicine* 95(10):491-497.

Levenson, L. J., C. Colenda, D. B. Larson, and J. C. Bareta. 1990. Methodology in consultation-liaison research: A classification of biases. *Psychosomatics* 31(4):367-375.

Maconochie, N., P. Doyle, G. Davies, S. Lewis, M. Pelerin, S. Prior, and P. Sampson. 2003. The study of reproductive outcome and the health of offspring of UK veterans of the Gulf War: Methods and description of the study population. *BMC Public Health* 3:4.

McCauley, L. A., S. K. Joos, P. S. Spencer, M. Lasarev, and T. Shuell. 1999. Strategies to assess validity of self-reported exposures during the Persian Gulf War. *Environmental Research* 81(3):195-205.

Murphy, D., R. Hooper, C. French, M. Jones, R. Rona, and S. Wessely. 2006. Is the increased reporting of symptomatic ill health in Gulf War veterans related to how one asks the question? *Journal of Psychosomatic Research* 61(2):181-186.

Murphy, D., M. Hotopf, and S. Wessely. 2008. Multiple vaccinations, health, and recall bias within UK armed forces deployed to Iraq: Cohort study. *British Medical Journal* 337:a220.

Ozakinci, G., W. K. Hallman, and H. M. Kipen. 2006. Persistence of symptoms in veterans of the first Gulf War: 5-year follow-up. *Environmental Health Perspectives* 114(10):1553-1557.

Pearce, N., H. Checkoway, and Kriebel D. 2007. Bias in occupational epidemiology studies. *Journal of Occupational and Environmental Medicine* 64:562-568.

Pierce, P. F. 1997. Physical and emotional health of Gulf War veteran women. *Aviation Space and Environmental Medicine* 68(4):317-321.

Proctor, S. P., T. Heeren, R. F. White, J. Wolfe, M. S. Borgos, J. D. Davis, L. Pepper, R. Clapp, P. B. Sutker, J. J. Vasterling, and D. Ozonoff. 1998. Health status of Persian Gulf War veterans: Self-reported symptoms, environmental exposures and the effect of stress. *International Journal of Epidemiology* 27(6):1000-1010.

Roy, M. J., P. A. Koslowe, K. Kroenke, and C. Magruder. 1998. Signs, symptoms, and ill-defined conditions in Persian Gulf War veterans: Findings from the comprehensive clinical evaluation program. *Psychosomatic Medicine* 60(6):663-668.

Salamon, R., C. Verret, M. A. Jutand, M. Begassat, F. Laoudj, F. Conso, and P. Brochard. 2006. Health consequences of the first Persian Gulf War on French troops. *International Journal of Epidemiology* 35(2):479-487.

Simmons, R., N. Maconochie, and P. Doyle. 2004. Self-reported ill health in male UK Gulf War veterans: A retrospective cohort study. *BMC Public Health* 4:1-10.

Steele, L. 2000. Prevalence and patterns of Gulf War illness in Kansas veterans: Association of symptoms with characteristics of person, place, and time of military service. *American Journal of Epidemiology* 152(10):992-1002.

Stretch, R. H., P. D. Bliese, D. H. Marlowe, K. M. Wright, K. H. Knudson, and C. H. Hoover. 1995. Physical health symptomatology of Gulf War-era service personnel from the states of Pennsylvania and Hawaii. *Military Medicine* 160(3):131-136.

Szklo, M. 1998. Population-based cohort studies. *Epidemiologic Reviews* 20(1):81-90.

Unwin, C., N. Blatchley, W. Coker, S. Ferry, M. Hotopf, L. Hull, K. Ismail, I. Palmer, A. David, and S. Wessely. 1999. Health of UK servicemen who served in Persian Gulf War. *Lancet* 353(9148):169-178.

Unwin, C., M. Hotopf, L. Hull, K. Ismail, A. David, and S. Wessely. 2002. Women in the Persian Gulf: Lack of gender differences in long-term health effects of service in United Kingdom Armed Forces in the 1991 Persian Gulf War. *Military Medicine* 167(5):406-413.

Wolfe, J., S. P. Proctor, J. D. Davis, M. S. Borgos, and M. J. Friedman. 1998. Health symptoms reported by Persian Gulf War veterans two years after return. *American Journal of Industrial Medicine* 33(2):104-113.

4

FACTOR ANALYSIS AND ITS USE IN STUDIES OF SYMPTOMS IN GULF WAR VETERANS

Because of the large number of symptoms reported by 1990–1991 Gulf War veterans that are potentially associated with chronic multisymptom illness (CMI), and the absence of definitive diagnostic tests for the condition, statistical analysis of reported symptoms has been used to evaluate CMI-defining symptoms. The two most frequently used statistical methods have been factor analysis and cluster analysis. Researchers began using statistical analyses to evaluate whether symptoms found in Gulf War veterans might constitute a unique syndrome. This chapter provides a brief discussion of the types of analyses and summaries of the studies that identified symptom factors or symptom clusters. In some cases, the researchers used their findings to inform the development of a case definition, but factor analysis alone cannot create a case definition. Although the focus of this chapter is on the studies that used factor and cluster analyses, there is overlap with the symptom studies reviewed in Chapter 3 and the case-definition studies discussed in Chapter 5. For a more detailed description of the statistical analyses used in the studies discussed below, see Appendix A.

FACTOR ANALYSIS

Factor analysis is a statistical method for conducting structural analyses of datasets. Large numbers of quantitative observations or responses can be resolved into "distinct patterns of occurrence" (Forbes et al., 2004). The patterns that are derived in a factor-analytic model are referred to as factors (Kline, 2000). Each factor explains a portion of the variance in such a way that the first factor explains the greatest percentage of the variance and each successive factor accounts for decreasing percentages of the variance. "Factor scores" estimate people's relative levels (number or severity) of symptoms associated with each factor. A factor score combines a person's responses to items associated with the factor and corresponding weights that represent the strength of associations between individual items and the factor. A factor score is generated for each person and each factor; thus, if a four-factor solution is posited, each person will have four factor scores. In some factor-analytic methods, the estimated factors are allowed to correlate with each other. When that approach is used, the intercorrelations are referred to as factor correlations. The relative strength of the relationship between any individual item and a factor is expressed as its factor loading. Factor loadings are the weights used in calculating people's factor scores. Factor analysis can be exploratory or confirmatory. In a confirmatory factor analysis factor loadings are posited a priori, and the resulting hypothesis is submitted to statistical testing (Kline, 2000). Confirmatory factor analysis is appropriate only when there is some body of knowledge or theory regarding the factor structure. In addition, in confirmatory factor analysis, items typically load on only a single factor. Some of the studies use another exploratory method known as principal component analysis (see Appendix A).

The data for factor-analytic studies can be people's responses to a set of items or a list of symptoms with respect to their presence or absence and their severity. The items can be dichotomous (such as yes–no questions) or have more than two possible responses (such as never–sometimes–always questions). In the case of CMI, responses to both kinds of items have been used in factor analysis.

Investigators use the results of a factor analysis to posit a plausible factor structure; that is, they estimate patterns regarding, for example, how different symptoms are related to each other and to the derived factors. It is inappropriate (and misleading) to refer to factors as "emerging" from a factor analysis (Pett et al., 2003). Such terminology inaccurately implies that a "true" set of factors underlie the data and that the factor set needs only to be unearthed. Factor-analytic results are seldom unequivocal, and they are influenced by a series of analytic decisions made by the researcher. An editor's note accompanying the Kang et al. (2002) study (discussed later in this chapter) on factor analysis states: "Factor analysis is not completely objective; for example, there are no definite rules for selecting the appropriate number of factors . . . or rules for selecting from among the many possible methods of rotation. It is an empirical method."

Factor Analysis for Data Reduction

Factor analysis has been used in studies of Gulf War veterans, initially to see whether a unique "Gulf War syndrome" could be identified and later to inform case definitions of CMI. In attempting to reduce the amount of data that would be gathered (the large and varied number of symptoms), researchers used factor analysis so that a structure that would include substantially fewer factors than symptoms could be proposed.

Typically in CMI studies, a survey that includes many individual items or symptoms is administered. For example, a survey administered by Knoke et al. (2000) included 98 individual items or symptoms, but the factor-analytic results suggested a data structure of five factors. In that example, one factor included 27 symptoms. Factor scores estimate people's relative levels of given factors. By reducing large sets of symptom data into their structural components, factor analysis can simplify comparisons of symptoms that are potentially related to Gulf War deployment.

The application of the data-reduction capabilities of factor analysis has been attractive for the study of Gulf War veterans' symptoms, but, as will be discussed below, studies' findings have been inconsistent. Different studies have identified different numbers of factors and assigned different names to common groups of symptoms. Some lack of consistency in findings of factor-analytic studies is expected because of differences in methods and questionnaires and because of random variation. Furthermore, when factor analyses are conducted without an a priori hypothesis, the subjective labeling of factors can be controversial, so factor labels should be critically reviewed (Ismail and Lewis, 2006). The factors posited in a given study will depend on the statistical approach used in the factor analysis, including decisions about how factors are "extracted" and "rotated." In addition, researchers must subjectively assign a name that they believe represents the items of a factor. To compare studies, it is necessary to understand which symptoms were associated with each factor, rather than depending on the label that researchers assigned to each factor.

Factor Analysis for Case Definitions

Although factor-analytic studies have facilitated and clarified comparisons of symptom prevalence and severity in deployed and nondeployed people, they have been less useful in specifying a case definition of CMI. The results of factor analyses do not differentiate among groups of people and cannot create a case definition. That fact has been obscured because investigators often operationalize a case definition by dichotomizing factor scores obtained from a factor-analytic model. However, people do not have factors. As explained above, everyone will have a score on every factor, but dichotomization of factor scores to define a "case" is a postprocessing decision made by investigators and not a direct result of the factor-analytic model.

Factor analysis can be used to evaluate whether the structure of symptom data is different in different populations (such as deployed and nondeployed), but this is not the same question as whether populations have higher symptom levels or greater symptom severity. The unique question that can be asked in the context of a factor-analytic study is whether the factor structure varies among compared populations. That question is most appropriately posited as a formal statistical test, in which the probability of observing the differences between the factor structures in the samples is estimated under the null hypothesis that the factor structures are the same in the two populations. For example, Ismail and colleagues (1999) compared three UK military cohorts: veterans of the Bosnia conflict, those deployed to the Gulf War, and Gulf War veterans not deployed to the Gulf. In addition to applying exploratory factor analysis, the investigators used a particular application of confirmatory factor analyses for which they generated statistics to estimate the goodness of fit of the factor-analytic model. They also tested a series of three models with different constraints: (1) factor correlations are equal in Gulf War–deployed and era veterans, (2) correlations between factors and factor loadings are equal in the two groups, and (3) all parameters are equal. Those models provided a direct, thorough, and hypothesis-based test of whether the factor structure differed in the two groups. That the constrained models did not fit significantly better than the unconstrained model indicates congruence in factor structure in the Gulf War–deployed and Gulf War–era veterans. However, most of the studies of factor-structure differences have failed to test the hypothesis directly, and none has used structural equation models. Instead, investigators have commonly relied on hypotheses related to factor scores or on descriptive comparisons of factor scores, factor loadings, and factor correlations.

There are two ways of comparing factor scores. In one, factor scores are generated for all members of reference and comparison groups. The scores are derived on the basis of a single factor-analytic model. The scores of deployed and nondeployed persons are compared to ascertain whether the presence or severity of the symptoms that define a factor differ by deployment status. No comparison of factor structure is made, because a single modeled structure is used to generate all scores. The other approach is to conduct separate factor analyses in the reference and comparison groups, derive factor scores for everyone on the basis of both factor-analytic models, and then compare the resulting scores; this is not an accepted method of comparing factor structures.

The studies that have used factor analysis to investigate symptoms in Gulf War veterans have used several analytic strategies. Some studies used statistical testing of the hypothesis that the factor structures of deployed and nondeployed veteran populations are significantly different (that is, testing the null hypothesis that the structures are the same) (Ismail et al., 1999), as discussed below and in Chapter 3. Other studies relied exclusively on descriptive statistical techniques, such as correlations among factors, factor scores, or factor loadings (Doebbeling et al., 2000; Kang et al., 2002). Finally, a number of studies used "visual inspection" to discern differences between the factor structures of deployed and nondeployed groups (Knoke et al., 2000; Nisenbaum et al., 2004; Shapiro et al., 2002).

FACTOR-ANALYSIS STUDIES[1]

This section discusses studies that used factors to determine whether veterans' symptoms might constitute a new syndrome or are a variant of a known syndrome. The cohorts are described fully in Chapter 3, and the descriptions below are limited to the methods and results associated with the factor analyses. The studies are presented by cohort and in the same order as in Chapter 3 and are also listed in Table 4.1. Many researchers used the data collected from their studies to inform or develop case definitions, which are discussed in greater detail in Chapter 5.

Department of Veterans Affairs

The nationally representative Department of Veterans Affairs (VA) study searched for potential new syndromes through factor analysis (Kang et al., 2002). Data were from a sample of 15,000 deployed and 15,000 nondeployed active-duty, reserve, National Guard, and retired service members in all four branches. Through questionnaures, the authors inquired about 47 symptoms on a three-point ordinal scale. On the basis of judgments of factor interpretability, they chose a five-factor solution for the nondeployed and a six-factor solution for the deployed sample. By inspection, the investigators judged that the first five factors were "very similar" in the two groups. The six factors were fatigue and depression,[2] musculoskeletal and rheumatologic,[3] gastrointestinal,[4] pulmonary,[5] upper respiratory,[6] and neurologic.[7] However, the last factor extracted contained symptoms consistent with neurologic impairment in the Gulf War group but not the non–Gulf War group. It should be noted that each successive factor that is extracted in a factor analysis accounts for less of the variance than the previous one. In the deployed sample, the sixth factor, labeled neurologic impairment, accounted for only 3% of the total variance, compared with 79% for the first factor. The neurologic factor was not extracted in the nondeployed group but accounted for 4% of the variance. In the neurologic factor, four symptoms—loss of balance or dizziness, speech difficulty, blurred vision, and tremors or shaking—loaded for the deployed but not for the nondeployed group. The authors indicated that

---

[1]The descriptions of the factor-analytic studies have been summarized from previously published Institute of Medicine reports (IOM, 2006, 2010).

[2]Awakening tired and worn out; concentration and memory problems; excessive fatigue; fatigue more than 24 hours after exertion; feeling anxious, irritable, or upset; feeling depressed or blue; sleep difficulty; and sleepiness during daytime.

[3]Back pain or spasms, generalized muscle aches, joint aches, numbness in hands or feet, swelling in joints, and swelling in extremities.

[4]Constipation, diarrhea, nausea; reflux, heartburn, or indigestion; stomach or abdominal pain; and vomiting.

[5]Coughing, irregular heartbeat, shortness of breath, tightness in chest, and wheezing.

[6]Coughing, runny nose, sore throat, swollen glands, and trouble swallowing.

[7]Blurred vision, concentration or memory problems, irregular heartbeat, loss of balance or dizziness, speech difficulty, sudden loss of strength, tremors or shaking, excessive fatigue, and fatigue more than 24 hours after exertion.

a group of 277 deployed veterans (2.4%) and a group of 43 nondeployed veterans (0.45%) had all four of those symptoms.

The authors interpreted their findings as suggesting a possible neurologic syndrome related to Gulf War deployment that would require objective supporting clinical evidence. It is possible, however, that this is an overinterpretation of the data inasmuch as the factor accounts for a small amount of the total variance and the nonextracted sixth factor in the nondeployed group accounted for more variance than it did in the deployed group.

The Iowa Study

The Iowa study (Iowa Persian Gulf Study Group, 1997) grouped symptoms into categories suggestive of existing syndromes or disorders, such as fibromyalgia or depression. Its finding of a considerably higher prevalence of symptom groups suggestive of fibromyalgia, depression, and cognitive dysfunction in Gulf War veterans motivated the first applications of factor analysis to grouping and classifying veterans' symptoms. Several years later, the same team of Iowa investigators performed a factor analysis on the Iowa cohort (Doebbeling et al., 2000). They studied the frequency and severity of 137 self-reported symptoms in 1,896 Gulf War veterans and 1,799 era veterans. Doebbeling et al. (2000) applied factor analysis in a sample of veterans who had been deployed and in a sample of nondeployed era controls. The deployed sample was divided into a training sample and a validation sample to evaluate the reproducibility of the factor solution for the group. Comparisons were made by correlating both factor loadings and factor scores in the deployed vs nondeployed samples. The authors identified three symptom factors in deployed veterans in the derivative sample that accounted for 35% of the variance: somatic distress (joint stiffness, myalgia, polyarthralgia, numbness or tingling, headache, and nausea), psychologic distress (feeling nervous, worrying, feeling distant or cut off; depression; and anxiety), and panic (anxiety attacks; a racing, skipping, or pounding heart; attacks of chest pain or pressure; and attacks of sweating). The researchers also conducted factor analysis in the nondeployed group and found the same three factors, which accounted for 29% of the variance. The authors concluded that their analyses did not support the existence of a new syndrome.

Oregon and Washington Veteran Studies

Investigators studied clusters of unexplained symptoms in a study of Portland area veterans by creating a new case definition of unexplained illness. Cases were identified on the basis of meeting a threshold number and combination of symptoms (cognitive and psychologic, and musculoskeletal) and on the basis of the duration of fatigue. Veterans whose symptom clusters remained unexplained at clinical examination (after exclusion of established diagnoses) were defined as constituting cases. Controls were those who at the time of clinical examination had no history of case-defining symptoms during or after their service in the Gulf War (Bourdette et al., 2001; Storzbach et al., 2000). The researchers undertook a factor analysis and then re-examined 48 symptoms in a second factor analysis. Three factors—cognitive and psychologic, mixed somatic, and musculoskeletal—were retained for followup factor analysis and accounted for 34.2% of the common variance. The authors used their three-factor solution to test the validity of their a priori case definition, which was composed of 35 symptoms encompassing musculoskeletal pain, cognitive and psychologic changes, gastrointestinal complaints, skin or mucous membrane lesions, and unexplained fatigue (discussed in greater detail in Chapter 5).

There were two major findings when the researchers compared the three-factor solution with the a priori case definition of Gulf War unexplained illnesses. First, their three factors did not include any symptoms related to the gastrointestinal system, the skin, or mucous membranes. Second, three of the symptoms—numbness in fingers or toes, clumsiness, and dizziness—were not included in the case definition. A limitation of the case-control design eliminated the possibility of examining differences between deployed and nondeployed veterans in that the study population by definition comprised only Gulf War veterans.

United Kingdom Veteran Studies

University of Manchester Veteran Study

Cherry et al. (2001) extracted seven distinct factors on the basis of data collected in a large, population-based study of British Gulf War–era service members who answered 95 symptom questions. Deployed veterans—two random samples of Gulf War veterans (main and validation cohorts)—were compared with a stratified sample of service members who had not been deployed. The seven factors, which accounted for 48% of the variance, could be found in all three groups separately: psychologic (24 symptoms), peripheral (10 symptoms), neurologic (13 symptoms), respiratory (11 symptoms), gastrointestinal (six symptoms), concentration (10 symptoms), and appetite (five symptoms). Deployed veterans' mean factor scores[8] were significantly higher for five factors: psychologic, peripheral, respiratory, gastrointestinal, and concentration. No difference was found in the neurologic factor scores, and appetite factor scores were significantly lower in the nondeployed cohort. None of the factors was exclusive to Gulf War veterans, so the investigators concluded that their findings did not support the existence of a new syndrome (Cherry et al., 2001).

Guy's, King's, and St. Thomas's Schools of Medicine Studies

Ismail et al. (1999) applied factor analysis to a representative sample of 7,379 UK veterans who served in the Bosnia conflict, who were deployed to the Gulf War, and who were not deployed. The researchers extracted three factors, which they labeled as mood and cognition (headache, irritability or outbursts of anger, sleeping difficulties, feeling jumpy or easily startled, unrefreshing sleep, fatigue, feeling distant or cut off from others, forgetfulness, loss of concentration, avoiding doing things or situations, and distressing dreams); respiratory system (unable to breathe deeply enough, faster breathing than normal, feeling short of breath at rest, and wheezing); and peripheral nervous system (tingling in fingers and arms, tingling in legs and arms, and numbness or tingling in fingers or toes). The pattern of symptom reporting by Gulf War veterans differed little from that by Bosnia and nondeployed era comparison groups, although the Gulf War cohort reported a higher frequency of symptoms and greater symptom severity.

In addition to applying exploratory factor analysis, Ismail et al. (1999) used a particular application of confirmatory factor analyses (see Appendix A for more information). They tested a series of three models with different constraints and concluded that the factor structure did not differ significantly between the Gulf War–deployed and the Gulf War–era veterans.

---

[8]Mean factor scores were computed by adding the sum of mean symptom scores (0–21) for each symptom that loaded onto the factor and dividing by the number of symptoms.

The UK authors interpreted their results as arguing against the existence of a unique Gulf War syndrome. Strengths of the study were its two comparison groups and its evaluation of the fit of the three-factor solution in the Bosnia and nondeployed cohort samples. The response rate of 65% may have introduced selection bias.

Using two previously studied cohorts (Fukuda et al., 1998; Ismail et al., 1999), Nisenbaum et al. (2004) conducted a factor analysis of symptom data on 3,454 UK Gulf War veterans, 1,979 people deployed to Bosnia for UN peacekeeping operations, and 2,577 nondeployed era veterans. The researchers also compared results with those on a sample of 1,163 US Gulf War veterans, but these comparisons were limited by the fact that the US sample responded to a different survey. On the basis of visual inspection of results, the investigators observed considerable overlap in factor structure and some differences. They judged the findings not to "represent a unique illness or 'Gulf War syndrome.'"

Australian Cohort

In a population-based study of all Australian Gulf War veterans, Forbes et al. (2004) applied factor analysis to findings from a 62-item symptom questionnaire that included measures of severity ("none," "mild," "moderate," and "severe"). They found three factors that accounted for 47.1% of the variance: psychophysiologic distress (23 symptoms), cognitive distress (20 symptoms), and arthroneuromuscular distress (6 symptoms). Those were broadly similar to factors extracted in previous analyses and were the same as factors that were based on data collected from a sample of nondeployed Australian veterans. However, although the prevalence was similar among deployed and nondeployed veterans, factor scores were higher among the deployed than among the nondeployed; the authors noted that this indicated a greater severity of symptoms. They concluded that there was no evidence of a unique pattern of self-reported symptoms in deployed veterans.

Seabee Studies

Haley et al. (1997) studied a battalion of 249 naval reservists called to active duty for the Gulf War. More than half the battalion had left the military by the time of the study; 41% of the battalion participated in the study. Of those participating, 70% reported having had a serious health problem since returning from the Gulf War. The study was the first to examine groupings of symptoms in Gulf War veterans with factor analysis. Through standardized symptom questionnaires and a two-stage exploratory factor analysis, the investigators defined what they considered to be either six syndromes or six variants of a single syndrome, which they labeled impaired cognition, confusion–ataxia, arthromyoneuropathy, phobia–apraxia, fever–adenopathy, and weakness–incontinence. One-fourth of the veterans in the study (63) were classified as having one of the six syndromes. The study was limited by its lack of a comparison group; the authors were unable to comment on the uniqueness of the factors in relation to other groups of veterans. Haley et al. (2001) attempted to replicate their factor-analysis findings in a validation cohort, which was separate from their original cohort of Seabees. The validation cohort of 335 consisted of veterans who were living in north Texas and who had registered with a VA clinic in Dallas or were recruited by advertising.

In the 2001 study, a more detailed questionnaire was used than in the earlier Seabee cohort in an effort to replicate the 1997 findings. Haley et al. (2001) undertook a series of analyses to test whether the factor structure that they found in the earlier cohort could be replicated in the larger and more representative cohort. In their confirmatory factor analysis, they imposed an additional constraint by allowing only four symptoms per factor for each of five models and compared the results of the five models with their earlier findings by using structure-equation models. The five models had either 12 or 16 measured variables, which loaded onto three first-order factors and zero or one higher-order factor. In two models, the four additional variables (or symptom factors) were allowed to load onto the primary or higher-order factors. The three primary syndrome factors were impaired cognition, confusion–ataxia, and central pain (termed arthromyoneuropathy in the original study); and the four additional variables or secondary symptom factors were chronic watery diarrhea, chronic fatigue involving excessive muscle weakness, chronic fever and night sweats, and middle and terminal insomnia. The higher-order factor was the presence of an underlying single Gulf War syndrome posited to explain all variance and covariance among the three first-order factors. Overall, 29% of participants had one or more of the three first-order factors, defined by dichotomizing the syndrome factor scale at 1.5, as in the original study. Haley et al. (2001) interpreted the results as confirming a three-factor solution, originally extracted in the Seabee cohort (Model 1). They also concluded that the three syndrome factors probably represented a higher-order syndrome, such as a single Gulf War syndrome, and that some additional symptoms (the four secondary symptom factors) appeared in all three syndrome variants. The researchers suggested that the confusion–ataxia syndrome may represent a more severe form of a single Gulf War syndrome of which impaired cognition and central pain variants (the other two syndrome factors) were less severe forms.

Knoke et al. (2000) applied factor analysis to data from a population of active-duty Seabees in response to the factor analysis conducted by Haley et al. (1997). The study population was drawn from US Navy construction-battalion personnel (Seabees) who were on active duty in 1990 and remained on active duty in 1994, when the study was conducted. The instrument contained 98 symptom questions. Among the 524 Gulf War veterans and 935 nondeployed Seabees, Knoke et al. (2000) performed three factor analyses: the first on the deployed Seabees, the second on the nondeployed Seabees, and the third on both. The three factor analyses accounted for 80%, 89%, and 93% of the total variance, and each extracted five factors. The factors were labeled insecurity or minor depression (27 symptoms), somatization (13 symptoms), depression (10 symptoms), obsessive-compulsive (7 symptoms), and malaise (7 symptoms). Knoke et al. (2000) derived standardized factor scores that were based on each solution and then evaluated whether the scores differed. Scores among the three analyses were similar for insecurity or minor depression; higher in Gulf War veterans for somatization, depression, and obsessive–compulsive; and higher in nondeployed Seabees for malaise.[9] Somatization, depression, and obsessive–compulsive affected an excess of about 20% of Gulf War veterans. This indirect method of testing the differences in factor structure led them to conclude that deployed and nondeployed veterans report "more of the same symptoms and illnesses" and that "identifying a new syndrome such as the putative Gulf War syndrome is a difficult task and is unlikely to be accomplished by factor analysis, or any other statistical methodology, performed on a small, selected group of Gulf War Veterans." The authors also conducted a discriminant analysis to test the ability of the factors to discriminate between Gulf War–deployed and nondeployed veterans: the probability of misclassification was 7.4% in nondeployed veterans and 76.5% in Gulf War–deployed veterans. The findings were similar to those of Doebbeling et

[9]Factor scores used to compare the groups were computed from the regression coefficients of the Gulf War veteran factor analysis, standardized for both groups by subtracting the median and dividing by the semi-interquartile range of the score for the Gulf War veteran group.

al. (2000), Fukuda et al. (1998), and Ismail et al. (1999). They concluded that there was no evidence of a unique spectrum of neurologic injury. Iannacchione et al. (2011) conducted a validation study of the Haley et al. (1997) case definition in a larger population of Gulf War veterans. The study is discussed in Chapter 5.

Pennsylvania Air National Guard Study

In response to a request from the Department of Defense, VA, and Pennsylvania, Fukuda et al. (1998) used factor analysis and other methods to assess the health status of Gulf War Air Force veterans. The objective was to assess the prevalence and causes of an unexplained illness in members of one Air National Guard unit compared with three comparison Air Force units. The investigators aimed to organize symptoms into a case definition and to carry out clinical evaluations of members of an Air National Guard unit (the index unit). They administered a 35-item symptom inventory that included symptom severity (mild, moderate, or severe) and duration (less than 6 months or 6 months or longer) and divided the 3,255 participants who had answered all symptom questions into two subsamples of 1,631 and 1,624. The authors conducted a principal components analysis of the first subsample, extracting 10 components with eigenvalues[10] greater than 1.0; three of the components accounted for 39.1% of the total variance. (See Appendix A for a discussion of the relationship between principal components analysis and factor analysis.) When the three components were examined in a confirmatory factor analysis in the second subsample, two were confirmed. The first, labeled mood–cognition–fatigue, consisted of these symptoms: feeling depressed, feeling anxious, feeling moody, difficulty in remembering or concentrating, trouble in finding words, difficulty in sleeping, and fatigue. The second, labeled musculoskeletal, consisted of these symptoms: joint stiffness, joint pain, and muscle pain. Fukuda et al. (1998) used 10 symptoms associated with the two factors from their confirmatory factor analysis to develop a preliminary case definition.

Department of Veterans Affairs Gulf War Health Registry

Hallman et al. (2003) examined patterns of reported symptoms in participants in the VA Gulf War Health Registry. The study sample consisted of a state-based random sample of 2,011 veteran registry members who resided in Delaware, Illinois, New Jersey, New York, North Carolina, Ohio, or Pennsylvania and who were not participating in other studies. Questionnaires included 48 symptoms, which were rated on a three-point ordinal scale, and were returned by 1,161 veterans (58% of the sample). The investigators divided the participants into two groups and conducted five factor analyses in each group to examine replicability. They identified four factors that accounted for 50.2% of the variance. The factors were mood–memory–fatigue (depression, anxiety, sudden mood changes, problems in concentrating and remembering, unexplained weakness, sleep problems, and unexplained fatigue); musculoskeletal (pain or numbness in joints or muscles); gastrointestinal (abdominal pain and gas, diarrhea, nausea, and vomiting); and throat and breathing (difficulty in swallowing, swollen glands, nose or sinus problems, coughing, difficulty in breathing, and difficulty in tasting). Like Cherry et al. (2001), Hallman et al. (2003) conducted a cluster analysis (see below) to examine consistency between the two statistical methods. The principal limitation of the study is the lack of a nondeployed

---

[10]In the context of factor analysis, an eigenvalue is a measure of variance. It indicates the amount of variation in the dataset that is accounted for by each factor. The eigenvalue for a given factor is the sum of the squared loadings of each variable on that factor (Ismail et al., 1999).

control group, which limits its ability to identify factors that may have been peculiar to exposure in the Gulf War. By starting with presumably the most symptomatic subset of Gulf War veterans (those who had left the service and registered with the Gulf War Health Registry), the authors might have had the chance of identifying clusters unique to Gulf War veterans if they existed. However, the four factors that they identified were largely similar to factors identified by other Gulf War investigators (Fukuda et al., 1998).

CLUSTER-ANALYSIS STUDIES

Another data-reduction technique used by Gulf War investigators is cluster analysis. This technique has been used in three cohorts to determine how groups of patients who have particular symptoms may be related to one another (Cherry et al., 2001; Everitt et al., 2002; Hallman et al., 2003). Cluster-analysis methods are discussed in Appendix A. In brief, cluster analysis posits a set number of clusters (groups of people) and then finds a solution that assigns people to clusters in such a way as to minimize the distances between people within clusters on the basis of their symptoms. There are several methods of cluster analysis, but all studies discussed use k-means cluster analysis methods (see Appendix A).

United Kingdom Veteran Studies

Several groups of researchers have examined symptoms in UK veterans. Two conducted cluster analyses.

University of Manchester Veteran Study

Cherry et al. (2001) sequentially partitioned members of three cohorts (Gulf War deployed, a second group of Gulf War deployed for validation purposes, and nondeployed) by using scores on 95 symptoms reported on a visual analogue scale. The authors stated that they chose the number of clusters to fit "by eye," choosing the largest number of clusters (six) when the clusters appeared to be similar among the three cohorts. In doing so, the authors precluded finding a Gulf War–specific cluster. Rather than showing the symptom means for each of the six clusters, they showed means by cluster of seven factor scores, which they had derived from a factor analysis of the same 95 symptoms, thus complicating the interpretation of the cluster analysis. Cluster 1 was composed primarily of well people and had a smaller proportion of Gulf War veterans (36.4%) than of nondeployed veterans (48.5%). Clusters 2 and 3 had similar prevalences in deployed and nondeployed groups. The final three clusters accounted for 23.8% of Gulf War veterans but only 9.8% of nondeployed veterans and included clusters with high scores on respiratory and gastrointestinal illnesses (cluster 4), on psychologic ill health (cluster 5), and both overall and especially on neurologic symptoms (cluster 6). There was an excess of 14% of Gulf War veterans in the three least healthy clusters.

Guy's, King's, and St. Thomas's Schools of Medicine Studies

Everitt et al. (2002) randomly sampled 500 participants from among three cohorts: Gulf War veterans, Bosnia veterans, and nondeployed Gulf War–era controls. They regrouped the original 50 "nonspecific symptoms common in the general population," which were then recategorized into 10 groups by body system with the same four-point severity score. They also used a technique, known as the gap statistic, that can be used to suggest the number of clusters that describe the data best (Tibshirani et al., 2001). The researchers identified five clusters by using cluster analysis. Inspection of the five-cluster solution shows clusters that display increasing severity of symptoms rather than distinct patterns of co-occurrences. Cluster 1 had low scores on all symptoms, cluster 2 had the highest scores on musculoskeletal symptoms and high scores on neuropsychologic, cluster 3 had high scores on neuropsychologic and higher scores on the remaining nine symptom groups, cluster 4 had high scores only on musculoskeletal symptoms, and cluster 5 had high scores on all 10 symptom groups, especially musculoskeletal and neuropsychologic. Many more Gulf War veterans fell into clusters 2, 3, and 5 than Bosnia or nondeployed veterans. With the gap statistic, two clusters were identified: one with low scores on each symptom group and one with higher mean scores on the musculoskeletal and neuropsychologic groups. This analysis also assessed the relationships between cluster membership and other variables; only cohort membership was significantly associated with cluster membership. Some 72% of Gulf War veterans, 87% of Bosnia veterans, and 94% of era-deployed veterans were classified in cluster 1. The authors interpreted their findings to mean that there was no convincing evidence of a Gulf War syndrome. Because groups of 10 symptoms rather than individual symptoms were used for the analysis, the contribution of individual symptoms to cluster formation is unknown.

Department of Veterans Affairs Gulf War Health Registry

Hallman et al. (2003) conducted cluster analysis in their examination of 1,161 veterans who were participating in the VA Gulf War Health Registry. The researchers used the mean factor scores from their factor analysis to group respondents on the basis of severity of symptoms. Examining the two randomly divided subsamples five times each but using cluster analysis, they identified two stable clusters. Cluster 1, making up 60.4% of the sample, consisted of veterans who reported no or mild symptoms in each of the four factors. Cluster 2, the remaining 39.6% of participants, consisted of veterans who had moderate to severe factor scores in the mood–memory–fatigue and musculoskeletal factors and mild to moderate scores in the gastrointestinal and throat and breathing factors. People classified in cluster 2 reported twice as many symptoms (37.2% vs 17.8%) as and reported more severe problems, were in poorer health, and had a greater reduction in mean activity than people in cluster 1.

SUMMARY AND CONCLUSIONS

The studies described in this chapter, despite their methodologic differences, have findings that are similar, that is, similar groups of symptoms were identified as falling roughly into factors associated with fatigue, pain, and neurocognitive symptoms (see Table 4.1). Less commonly reported are factors that involve gastrointestinal and respiratory symptoms. Taken together, the studies' findings do not support a unique syndrome, although they do highlight more frequent and severe symptoms in Gulf War–deployed than in nondeployed.

Well-conducted factor analyses should have high participation rates and include representative samples. Some of the studies fall short on those two criteria. For example, several studies included members of only one branch of service (Fukuda et al., 1998; Haley et al., 1997; Knoke et al., 2000), collected small samples (Haley et al., 1997), or drew samples only from symptomatic groups of veterans (Haley et al., 1997; Hallman et al., 2003). Another problem is the lack of a comparison group in some of the studies, which limits investigators' ability to compare factor structure in deployed and other groups (such as nondeployed and deployed elsewhere) (Bourdette et al., 2001; Haley et al., 1997). Although results of those studies are valuable and add rich detail to the epidemiologic literature surrounding Gulf War veterans, other studies are more representative, and their results therefore more generalizable (Cherry et al., 2001; Doebbeling et al., 2000; Ismail et al., 1999; Kang et al., 2002). Findings of the more representative studies were quite similar, broadly describing neurologic, psychologic, cognitive, fatigue, and musculoskeletal symptoms. One exception to the congruence of those findings is the extraction by Kang et al. (2002) of factors that represented symptoms labeled as gastrointestinal, pulmonary, and upper respiratory.

Three studies compared factors in representative deployed and nondeployed groups (Cherry et al., 2001; Doebbeling et al., 2000; Ismail et al., 1999). The factors extracted in those studies were remarkably similar between the deployed and nondeployed groups, and the findings did not suggest a unique complex of symptoms in the deployed group. In each of the studies, as in many of the less generalizable studies, symptoms were more frequent and more severe (in papers that reported severity) in the deployed than in the nondeployed groups. The three studies that used cluster analysis had broadly similar findings. The two studies that included nondeployed comparison groups (Cherry et al., 2001; Everitt et al., 2002) failed to identify a cluster of people that presented with a unique syndrome. Each study identified a highly symptomatic cluster of people that contained a higher proportion of Gulf War veterans than of non–Gulf War veterans, ranging from 14% in Cherry et al. (2001) to 22.2% in Everitt et al. (2002). The cluster analyses were consistent with the findings of the most representative factor-analysis studies: although they did not support a unique symptom complex in Gulf War veterans, they found that these veterans were more symptomatic than their nondeployed counterparts.

Factor analysis and cluster analysis may be useful methods for making sense of the large number of symptoms potentially associated with CMI. However, the findings obtained with these methods must be validated against other observed variables. The choice of variables to include in a model is critical, and omission of key symptoms will result in models that do not capture the most salient features of CMI. In most of the studies, the percentage of variance explained is not great. The heterogeneity of the survey questions makes it difficult to account for a lot of the variance with only a few factors. Moreover, the validity of factor analysis or cluster analysis depends on the quality of data. Methodologic flaws in such studies can bias their results (Ismail and Lewis, 2006). The committee notes that neither factor analysis nor cluster analysis alone can directly produce a case definition; such definitions are the product of postprocessing of factor-analytic model results (for example, dichotomization of factor scores to operationalize a case definition).

Given the historical dependence on factor-analytic methods in CMI studies and the methodologic flaws associated with many of them, the following are suggested practices for future factor-analytic studies. More details and definitions are available in Appendix A. For interested readers, excellent published resources provide systematic and extensive descriptions of factor-analytic methods; see, for example, Brown et al. (2012), Kline (2000), Norman and Streiner (2003), Pett et al. (2003), Rummel (1970), and Stewart (1981).

- Describe the factor-analytic process in sufficient detail to allow replication, including the wording of each item, the methods used to decide the number of factors, the method of factor extraction, the method of factor rotation, and any additional postprocessing conducted by the authors.
- Because factor analysis is a family of methods rather than a single method, select a factor-analytic approach that is aligned with the research question.

- In deciding how many factors to extract in an exploratory factor analysis, consider parallel analysis—a simulation-based approach in which factors are retained only if their eigenvalues exceed what would be obtained in random samples with no underlying factors.
- Factor analysis is not ideal for application to dichotomous (such as yes–no) data, so symptom survey items should include multiple response categories for collecting symptom data.
- Account for the measurement level of the data when conducting factor analysis; for example, use a polychoric correlation matrix, rather than a Pearson correlation matrix, to account for ordinal-level data. See Appendix A for further discussion of these matrices.
- Select a factor rotation method that is consistent with expectations regarding the relationships among factors (for example, choose an oblique rotation when factors are expected to correlate with each other).
- Explicitly test whether factor-analytic results are reproducible (for example, compare with a "holdout" sample and replicate in an independent sample).
- Apply a confirmatory factor model only when there is an a priori hypothesis regarding data structure.
- To evaluate whether the factor structure of symptom data differs in different populations (for example, in deployed vs nondeployed), posit and test the question as a formal statistical hypothesis.

TABLE 4.1 Factor Analyses of Gulf War Veteran Cohorts

Reference	Population	Variables and Data	Method	Rotation[a]	No. Factors Isolated; % Variance Explained	Factors Identified	Unique Factors in GWVs?
Kang et al., 2002	Active and retired, n = 19,383	Ordinal; 47 symptoms coded as 0 = none, 1 = mild, or 2 = severe.	Iterative principal-factor analysis	Oblique	6; % not reported	Fatigue or depression, neurologic, musculoskeletal–rheumatologic, gastrointestinal, pulmonary, and upper respiratory	Factors similar, but 4 neurologic symptoms loaded on neurologic factor for deployed but not nondeployed.
Doebbeling et al., 2000	Active and reserve, n = 3,695	Ordinal and dichotomous; 78 symptoms rated 0 (not present) to 4 (extremely bothersome).	Unknown	Orthogonal and oblique	3; 35% in deployed, 30% in nondeployed	Somatic distress, psychologic distress, and panic	Correlation between derivative and validation samples; same factors in nondeployed. Prevalence not stated.
Bourdette et al., 2001	Active and reserve, n = 443	Dichotomous; 69 symptoms; response scale not reported.	PCA	Orthogonal	3; 34.2%	Cognitive–psychologic, mixed somatic, and musculoskeletal	NA
Cherry et al., 2001	Active and retired, n = 11,914	Interval; 95 symptoms; visual analogue symptom scores from 1 to 21.	PCA separately in 3 cohorts: Gulf War–deployed (main), Gulf War–deployed (holdout or validation sample), and not deployed	Orthogonal	7; 48%	Psychologic, peripheral, neurologic, respiratory, gastrointestinal, concentration, and appetite	All present; mean factor scores higher in GWVs for psychologic, peripheral, respiratory, gastrointestinal, concentration; lower for appetite.

Reference	Population	Variables and Data	Method	Rotation[a]	No. Factors Isolated; % Variance Explained	Factors Identified	Unique Factors in GWVs?
Ismail et al., 1999	Active, n = 3,214	Ordinal and dichotomous; 50–52 nonspecific symptoms rated as absent, mild, moderate, or severe; cases with missing responses were excluded.	Principal factors	Orthagonal	3; ~20%	Mood–cognition, respiratory system, and peripheral nervous system	No, but 3-factor solution fit less well in Bosnian cohort than in GW-deployed and less well in nondeployed than in Bosnian cohort. Prevalence not mentioned.
Nissenbaum et al., 2004	UK GW veterns, n = 3,454; UK Bosnia-deployed, n = 1,979; US GW veterans, n = 1,163	Dichotomous; 50 symptoms; scored yes or no; symptoms differed between US and UK cohorts.	Exploratory factor analysis; confirmatory factor analysis	Othogonal	3; % not reported	Respiratory, mood–cognition, and peripheral nervous	Gastrointestinal symptom factor appeared in UK GW veteran data; musculoskeletal factor appeared in US GW veteran data.
Forbes et al., 2004	Active and retired, n = 2,781	Ordinal; 63 symptoms ranked by severity (none, mild, moderate, or severe); reduced to 62 because of low prevalence (seizures in preceding month); 28 items recoded from 4 to 3 categories; 25 to 2 categories.	Unknown	Orthogonal and oblique	3; 47.1%	Psychophysiologic distress, cognitive distress, and arthroneuromuscular distress	No. Prevalence similar but severity higher in GWVs.

Reference	Population	Variables and Data	Method	Rotation[a]	No. Factors Isolated; % Variance Explained	Factors Identified	Unique Factors in GWVs?
Haley et al., 1997	Active and retired (Navy), n = 249	Interval.	Principal-axis factor analysis[a]	Orthogonal and oblique	6; 71%	Impaired cognition, confusion–ataxia, and arthromyoneuropathy, phobia–apraxia, fever–adenopathy, and weakness–incontinence	NA
Haley et al., 2001	Active, reserve, retired, n = 335	Continuous.	Principal factors (in developmental sample)	Orthogonal and oblique	Forced into 5 models with 3 syndrome factors; 29%	Impaired cognition, confusion–ataxia, and central pain	Compared fit of factor analysis with that found in Haley et al. (1997) by using structural estimating equations. Some models also fitted higher-order factor "Gulf War syndrome" and loaded 4 additional symptoms (chronic fatigue involving excessive muscle weakness, chronic fever and night sweats, middle and terminal insomnia, and chronic watery diarrhea) onto higher-order factor.
Knoke et al., 2000	Active (Navy), n = 1,459	Ordinal and dichotomous; 98 symptoms.	Principal-axis factor analysis[b]	Orthogonal	5; 80-93%	Insecurity, somatization, depression; obsessive–compulsive; and malaise	Somatization, depression, obsessive–compulsive. 3 times as common in GWVs vs NDVs.

Reference	Population	Variables and Data	Method	Rotation[a]	No. Factors Isolated; % Variance Explained	Factors Identified	Unique Factors in GWVs?
Fukuda et al., 1998	Active and reserve (Air Force), n = 3,255	Ordinal; 35 symptoms, including severity (mild, moderate, or severe) and duration (<6 months or ≥6 months).	PCA followed by confirmatory factor analysis	Oblique	3; 39.1%	Fatigue, mood–cognition, and musculoskeletal pain	45% of deployed met factor score–based case definition of CMI vs 15% of nondeployed.
Hallman et al., 2003	Retired, participants in VA Gulf War Health Registry who felt their illness was service-related, n = 981	Ordinal; 48 symptoms; present or recurring, mild, moderate, or severe. Data split into halves.	Principal-axis factor analysis[b]	Oblique	4; 50.2%	Mood–memory–fatigue, musculoskeletal, gastrointestinal, and throat–breathing	

NOTE: CMI = chronic multisymptom illness; GW = Gulf War; GWV = Gulf War veteran; NDV = nondeployed veteran; PCA = principal components analysis.

[a]Factor solutions are rotated to maximize high loadings and minimize low loadings. *Orthogonal* rotation algorithms extract factors so that they do not correlate with one another. *Oblique* rotation algorithms allow factors to correlate with one another.

[b]Principal-axis factor analysis is a common kind of factor analysis.

REFERENCES

Bourdette, D. N., L. A. McCauley, A. Barkhuizen, W. Johnston, M. Wynn, S. K. Joos, D. Storzbach, T. Shuell, and D. Sticker. 2001. Symptom factor analysis, clinical findings, and functional status in a population-based case control study of Gulf War unexplained illness. *Journal of Occupational and Environmental Medicine* 43(12):1026-1040.

Brown, B. L., S. G. Hendrix, D. W. Hedges, and T. B. Smith. 2012. *Multivariate Analysis for the Biobeahvioral and Social Sciences: A Graphical Approach*. Hoboken, NJ: John Wiley and Sons, Inc.

Cherry, N., F. Creed, A. Silman, G. Dunn, D. Baxter, J. Smedley, S. Taylor, and G. J. Macfarlane. 2001. Health and exposures of united kingdom Gulf War veterans. Part II: The relation of health to exposure. *Journal of Occupational and Environmental Medicine* 58(5):299-306.

Doebbeling, B. N., W. R. Clarke, D. Watson, J. C. Torner, R. F. Woolson, M. D. Voelker, D. H. Barrett, and D. A. Schwartz. 2000. Is there a Persian Gulf War syndrome? Evidence from a large population-based survey of veterans and nondeployed controls. *American Journal of Medicine* 108(9):695-704.

Everitt, B., K. Ismail, A. S. David, and S. Wessely. 2002. Searching for a Gulf War syndrome using cluster analysis. *Psychological Medicine* 32(8):1371-1378.

Forbes, A. B., D. P. McKenzie, A. J. Mackinnon, H. L. Kelsall, A. C. McFarlane, J. F. Ikin, D. C. Glass, and M. R. Sim. 2004. The health of Australian veterans of the 1991 Gulf War: Factor analysis of self-reported symptoms. *Journal of Occupational and Environmental Medicine* 61(12):1014-1020.

Fukuda, K., R. Nisenbaum, G. Stewart, W. W. Thompson, L. Robin, R. M. Washko, D. L. Noah, D. H. Barrett, B. Randall, B. L. Herwaldt, A. C. Mawle, and W. C. Reeves. 1998. Chronic multisymptom illness affecting Air Force veterans of the Gulf War. *Journal of the American Medical Association* 280(11):981-988.

Haley, R. W., T. L. Kurt, and J. Hom. 1997. Is there a Gulf War syndrome? Searching for syndromes by factor analysis of symptoms. *Journal of the American Medical Association* 277(3):215-222. [Erratum appears in *Journal of the American Medical Association* 1997; 278(5):388.]

Haley, R. W., G. D. Luk, and F. Petty. 2001. Use of structural equation modeling to test the construct validity of a case definition of Gulf War syndrome: Invariance over developmental and validation samples, service branches and publicity. *Psychiatry Research* 102(2):175-200.

Hallman, W. K., H. M. Kipen, M. Diefenbach, K. Boyd, H. Kang, H. Leventhal, and D. Wartenberg. 2003. Symptom patterns among Gulf War registry veterans. *American Journal of Public Health* 93(4):624-630.

Iannacchione, V. G., J. A. Dever, C. M. Bann, K. A. Considine, D. Creel, C. P. Carson, H. Best, and R. W. Haley. 2011. Validation of a research case definition of Gulf War illness in the 1991 US military population. *Neuroepidemiology* 37(2):129-140.

IOM (Institute of Medicine). 2006. *Gulf War and Health, Volume 4: Health Effects of Serving in the Gulf War*. Washington, DC: The National Academies Press.

IOM. 2010. *Gulf War and Health, Volume 8: Update of Health Effects of Serving in the Gulf War*. Washington, DC: The National Academies Press.

Iowa Persian Gulf Study Group. 1997. Self-reported illness and health status among Gulf War veterans: A population-based study. *Journal of the American Medical Association* 277(3):238-245.

Ismail, K., and G. Lewis. 2006. Multi-symptom illnesses, unexplained illness and Gulf War syndrome. *Philosophical Transactions of the Royal Society B: Biological Sciences* 361(1468):543-551.

Ismail, K., B. Everitt, N. Blatchley, L. Hull, C. Unwin, A. David, and S. Wessely. 1999. Is there a Gulf War syndrome? *Lancet* 353(9148):179-182.

Kang, H. K., C. M. Mahan, K. Y. Lee, F. M. Murphy, S. J. Simmens, H. A. Young, and P. H. Levine. 2002. Evidence for a deployment-related Gulf War syndrome by factor analysis. *Archives of Environmental Health* 57(1):61-68.

Kline, P. 2000. *The Handbook of Psychological Testing, Second Edition*. New York: Routledge.

Knoke, J. D., T. C. Smith, G. C. Gray, K. S. Kaiser, and A. W. Hawksworth. 2000. Factor analysis of self-reported symptoms: Does it identify a Gulf War syndrome? *American Journal of Epidemiology* 152(4):379-388.

Nisenbaum, R., K. Ismail, S. Wessely, C. Unwin, L. Hull, and W. C. Reeves. 2004. Dichotomous factor analysis of symptoms reported by UK and US veterans of the 1991 Gulf War. *Population Health Metrics* 2.

Norman, G. R., and D. L. Streiner. 2003. *PDQ Statistics, Third Edition*. BC Decker Inc. http://www.amazon.com/Pdq-Statistics-Series-Third-Edition/dp/1550092073 (accessed October 6, 2013).

Pett, M. A., N. R. Lackey, and J. J. Sullivan. 2003. *Making Sense of Factor Analysis: The Use of Factor Analysis for Instrument Development in Health Care Research*. Thousand Oaks, CA: Sage Publications.

Rummel, R. J. 1970. *Applied Factor Analysis*. Evanston, IL: Northwestern University Press.

Shapiro, S. E., M. R. Lasarev, and L. McCauley. 2002. Factor analysis of Gulf War illness: What does it add to our understanding of possible health effects of deployment? *American Journal of Epidemiology* 156(6):578-585.

Stewart, D. W. 1981. The application and misapplication of factor analysis in marketing research. *Journal of Marketing Research* 18:51-62.

Storzbach, D., K. A. Campbell, L. M. Binder, L. McCauley, W. K. Anger, D. S. Rohlman, and C. A. Kovera. 2000. Psychological differences between veterans with and without Gulf War unexplained symptoms. Portland Environmental Hazards Research Center. *Psychosomatic Medicine* 62(5):726-735.

Tibshirani, R., G. Walther, and T. Hastie. 2001. Estimating the number of clusters in a data set via the gap statistic. *Journal of the Royal Statistical Society. Series B (Statistical Methodology)* 63(2):411-423.

5

CHRONIC MULTISYMPTOM ILLNESS CASE DEFINITIONS AND RECOMMENDATIONS

The Department of Veterans Affairs (VA) tasked the committee with determining whether one of several existing case definitions of chronic multisymptom illness (CMI) in Gulf War veterans is adequate, whether an existing case definition needs to be revised, or whether a new case definition needs to be established. At the committee's first meeting, VA representatives noted that "given the different case-definition criteria and different ways of evaluating symptoms, it has been difficult to compare research results among studies." They noted further that "consistent use of a case definition is necessary for advancing research." This chapter examines the current case definitions of CMI and proposes a way forward.

The committee recognizes the difficulty of establishing a consensus case definition of CMI, given the lack of uniform symptoms, the variety of symptoms, and the long onset and duration. However, CMI is an important cause of disability in Gulf War veterans and the lack of a consensus case definition poses problems for those who are suffering with it. The absence of a consensus case definition is a fundamental weakness of CMI research in that the lack of an agreed on case definition can make it difficult to identify cases and controls. It also prevents the accurate estimation of the burden of illness in the veteran population, the use of generalizable results, the accumulation of valid information about the condition, and the effectiveness of treatment.

In a clinical setting, the absence of an agreed upon case definition of CMI not only can result in considerable uncertainty about the diagnosis, but might limit the ability to select and administer effective treatments. Practically, that means that there will be veterans who incorrectly receive or do not receive a diagnosis of CMI and the prescribed course of treatments might not be helpful. Inappropriate treatment can have an adverse effect on the health of a veteran in connection with worry about the lack of improvement, possible side effects of treatment, and the cost of treatment. The impact on health care services may also be considerable, and whether treatment is an effective use of limited resources should be cause for concern.

For those reasons, the committee believes that supporting the development of a case definition or the adoption of a current definition will move the field forward. The committee recognizes that as the knowledge base changes, a case definition will need to evolve as has occurred in other symptom-based conditions, such as irritable bowel syndrome, chronic fatigue syndrome (CFS), and fibromyalgia.

EXISTING CASE DEFINITIONS

This section discusses the studies that have proposed case definitions of CMI in Gulf War veterans. The definitions have been informed by questionnaires and surveys used in cohort studies (see Chapter 3), statistical analyses (see Chapter 4), and clinical observations. Because of the wide array of symptoms found in 1990–1991 Gulf War veterans and the lack of definitive diagnostic tests, several case definitions have been proposed and used by various researchers, but no case definition has been universally accepted. Each definition is described below; details about how the cohorts were assembled can be found in Chapter 3 and are not presented here. Table 5.1 summarizes the definitions and may be found later in this chapter. It should be noted that the authors of the definitions discussed below do not address, nor did they intend to address, all the elements of a typical case definition (see Chapter 2). A standard set of criteria regarding time (a defined period of onset), place, exposures, and clinical and laboratory findings would have been useful; however, given the lag in time between first reports of illness and epidemiologic study, lack of exposure monitoring, and the absence of validated laboratory tests, it is not possible to define many of the typical elements associated with a case definition.

Haley and Colleagues

Haley et al. (1997) defined multisymptom illness in Gulf War veterans on the basis of factor analysis (see Chapter 4) and clinical observation by using two distinct populations. The factor analysis included 249 (41%) of the 606 Gulf War veterans of the Twenty-Fourth Reserve Naval Construction Battalion from five southeastern states. The study was the first to examine groupings of symptoms in Gulf War veterans by using factor analysis. Through standardized symptom questionnaires and a two-stage exploratory factor analysis, the investigators defined what they considered to be either six syndromes or six variants of a single syndrome, which they labeled impaired cognition, confusion–ataxia, arthromyoneuropathy, phobia–apraxia, fever–adenopathy, and weakness–incontinence. One fourth of the veterans in the study (63) were classified as having one of the six syndromes. On the basis of factor analysis and postprocessing decisions, the study defined three syndromes: impaired cognition, confusion–ataxia, and arthromyoneuropathy.

The clinical observation included selected cases from a Department of Defense (DOD) military survey and registry. In an effort to compare the factor-analysis–derived syndromes with clinical cases, the veterans in the DOD registry had to meet several criteria—a veteran must have served in the theater of operations during August 8, 1990–July 31, 1991; must not have had a physician's diagnosis of other medical and psychiatric illnesses that could cause symptoms; and must have experienced at least five of the following eight symptoms: fatigue; arthralgia or low back pain; headache; intermittent diarrhea without bloody stools; neuropsychiatric complaints of forgetfulness, difficulty concentrating, depression, memory loss, or easy irritability; difficulty sleeping; low-grade fever; and weight loss. The degree of association between the factor-analysis–derived syndromes and the clinical case definition was assessed with logistic regression analysis. When the clinical definition was compared with the factor-analysis–derived syndromes, it was found to be strongly associated with syndromes 1 and 3 (impaired cognition and arthromyoneuropathy). The clinical definition proposed by Haley et al. (1997) captured 34% (85) of the veterans, whereas the six-factor derived syndromes identified 25% of the veterans (5% as syndrome 1 and 9% as syndrome 3).

Haley et al. (2001) attempted to replicate their factor-analysis findings in a validation cohort, which was separate from their original cohort of Seabees. The validation cohort consisted of 335 veterans who were living in north Texas and had registered with a VA clinic in Dallas or were recruited by advertising. In comparison with the original Seabee cohort, participants in the validation cohort were more likely to have served in the Army and to be representative of those who served in the gulf with regard to racial and ethnic background, age, and wartime military status. The three primary syndrome factors were impaired cognition, confusion–ataxia, and central pain (termed arthromyoneuropathy in the original study); and the four additional variables or secondary symptom factors were chronic watery diarrhea, chronic fatigue involving excessive muscle weakness, chronic fever and night sweats, and middle and terminal insomnia. The higher-order factor was the presence of an underlying single Gulf War syndrome that could explain all variance and covariance among the three first-order factors. Overall, 29% of participants had one or more of the three first-order factors, defined by dichotomizing the syndrome factor scale at 1.5 standard deviations above the mean, as in the original study. The authors found that the apparent three-factor solution, originally demonstrated in the Seabee cohort, was also present in this new cohort (Model 1); that the three syndrome factors probably represented a higher-order syndrome, such as a single Gulf War syndrome (Model 2); and that some additional symptoms (the four secondary symptom factors) appeared in all three syndrome variants. They suggested that syndrome 3 (symptoms related to central pain) may not be a separate syndrome but may reflect a higher-order factor related to overall Gulf War syndrome. The authors concluded that the three-syndrome factor model is the only empirically developed and validated case definition available.

The small sample in the study may have limited exploration of less common symptoms, and the nonrandom nature of the sample may have limited to some degree the generalizability of some of the results, such as syndrome prevalence; but the detailed questionnaires and the external validation of the findings through comparison with the Seabee cohort were strengths of the second study. Note that this study, by design, had no comparison group. The authors were seeking to validate the presence of a symptom complex in deployed veterans rather than to examine its prevalence in deployed and nondeployed forces. They concluded by recommending a study of a national randomly selected sample of deployed and nondeployed Gulf War–era military populations with their methods of symptom measurement and syndrome definition.

To validate the definition posed by Haley et al. (2001), Iannacchione et al. (2011) conducted a study of a population-based sample of more than 8,000 of Gulf War–deployed and nondeployed (but fit for deployment) service personnel. The questionnaire, conducted in 2007–2009, contained questions about symptoms used to develop the syndromes found by Haley et al. (2001) and symptoms used for other case definitions—such as that of the Centers for Disease Control and Prevention (CDC)— and similar conditions, for example, CFS and fibromyalgia. The authors did not replicate the exploratory factor analysis. They used the factor weights from the original Haley et al. study to create factor scales and to determine which syndrome fit each person in the study, as was done in both earlier studies of the factor case definition (Haley et al., 1997, 2001). Results showed similar goodness-of-fit statistics for all three studies. Some 14% of the deployed and 4% of the nondeployed fit any of the six syndromes that make up the factor case definition.

Centers for Disease Control and Prevention

The CMI case definition developed by CDC was derived from clinical data and statistical analyses (Fukuda et al., 1998). The investigators conducted a cross-sectional survey in a Pennsylvania-based Air National Guard unit and three comparison Air Force units. Two case definitions were developed on the basis of clinical data and statistical analyses from a survey of 35 symptoms. To develop the clinical definition, the investigators required that the illness be chronic (6 months or longer) and be present 2.5 times more in deployed than in nondeployed veterans. The method identified symptoms of fatigue, difficulty remembering or concentrating, moodiness, difficulty sleeping, and joint pain or stiffness. The analytic approach included a principal-components analysis followed by a confirmatory factor analysis. The researchers considered the results to identify the same symptoms as in their clinical definition. Two factor-analytic definitions were developed: the factor-score approach, in which participants who had factors scores in the top 25th percentile were cases; and a symptom-category approach—based on the symptom groups identified in the factor analysis (categories of fatigue, mood–cognition, and musculoskeletal)—that specified that a case must have at least one symptom in each of at least two categories. Because there was a high degree of agreement between the two definitions on the basis of prevalence in the study population, the authors endorsed the symptom-category approach as more practical for a clinical setting.

The final case definition included an indicator of severity and was used in a clinical study that included clinical evaluation. The definition requires more than one chronic (≥6 months) symptom in each of at least two of three categories: fatigue, mood and cognition, and musculoskeletal. Severe cases were identified if at least one symptom in each of the required categories was rated as severe. Of 1,155 participating Gulf War veterans, 6% had severe CMI, and 39% had mild to moderate CMI; of the 2,520 nondeployed era veterans, 0.7% had severe and 14% had mild to moderate CMI. Risk factors associated with CMI were deployment to the Gulf War, rank, being female, age, and smoking; cases also reported reduced functioning. The definition has been used in numerous studies (discussed below) and fulfills many of the requirements for a case definition (Chapter 2). It also allows subclassification by severity.

Several followup studies of Gulf War veterans have used the CDC definition in other study populations, some with modifications. For example, Rayhan et al. (2013) used the CDC criteria in a clinical study of migraines; the researchers required that cases had been deployed to the Persian Gulf for at least 30 days and excluded participants who had chronic diseases that accounted for their CMI symptoms. Among the 50 CMI cases identified and 45 controls, the authors found that 64% of CMI cases had migraines (11 times more likely than controls to suffer from migraines).

Kelsall et al. (2009) conducted a study using a questionnaire and medical assessment of 2002 Australian veterans with a modified version of the CDC definition and incorporated results of an Australian factor analysis (Forbes et al., 2004). The Kelsall et al. study required that veterans had one or more symptoms in the preceding month with at least moderate severity from at least three of four categories: fatigue, psychophysiologic, cognitive, and arthroneuromuscular. Of the 1,381 Gulf War veterans who participated in the study, 25.6% met this definition of CMI, as did 16% of the 1,377 nondeployed era veterans. The study found that veterans who had CMI were also significantly more likely to suffer from psychiatric disorders, chronic fatigue, and reduced functional impairment and quality of life, but objective outcomes were similar in the two groups. Gulf War veterans who had CMI had more hospitalizations, obstructive liver disease, and Epstein-Barr virus exposure but were otherwise similar to nondeployed Gulf War–era veterans (Kelsall et al., 2009).

Other studies have used the CDC definition to assess cohorts longitudinally and describe potential risk factors. In a 10-year followup of a cross-sectional survey, 1,035 deployed and 1,116 nondeployed veterans who had participated in the 1995–1996 National Health Survey (studied by Fukuda et al., 1998) indicated that CMI was twice as likely in deployed as in nondeployed veterans. Results showed that 28.9% of deployed (7% severe) and 15.8% of nondeployed (1.6% severe) met the criteria for CMI. Both deployed and nondeployed participants who had CMI reported lower quality of life and more symptom-based medical conditions, metabolic syndrome, psychiatric disorders, prewar anxiety, and depression than those who did not have CMI. Deployed CMI veterans reported more nicotine dependence and infectious mononucleosis, but nondeployed CMI veterans reported more headaches and gastritis (Blanchard et al., 2006).

Hallman et al. (2003) conducted an exploratory factor analysis and cluster analysis among 1,161 participating veterans who resided in Delaware, Illinois, New Jersey, New York, North Carolina, Ohio, or Pennsylvania and compared results with the CDC case definition of CMI. Four factors were extracted in the factor analysis and were labeled mood/memory/fatigue, musculoskeletal, gastrointestinal, and throat/breathing, and severity was categorized by cluster analysis: group 1, mild or no problems; group 2, moderate to severe symptoms. Some 75% of group 1 and 100% of group 2 (all but one individual) met the CDC case definition. The study was not designed to be representative of US veterans; the investigators sought veterans who believed that they suffered from Gulf War–related illnesses. In a 5-year followup, Ozakinci et al. (2006) surveyed 390 veterans a second time. That study did not use a case definition, but it did distinguish between veterans (60%) reporting good health and no or few symptoms and those (40%) reporting fair or poor health and many symptoms (37 symptoms on the average). Ten years after the Gulf war, those who were highly symptomatic improved less and reported greater symptom severity than those who had had lesser symptomatology initially.

Wolfe et al. (2002) assessed 945 respondents from the Ft. Devens cohort in 1997–1998 by using the CDC case definition. Symptom onset must have occurred during or after the Gulf War and symptom frequency and severity were assessed, but a requirement for duration of more than 6 months could not be met, owing to lack of data. About 60% of respondents met the case definition of CMI, including 30% who had severe CMI. Important risk factors for CMI included being female, having less than a college education, being a reservist, and having a variety of deployment-related environmental exposures. The study did not include a comparison group and was composed entirely of Army personnel.

Unwin et al. (1999) assessed the health of and symptoms in more than 8,000 Gulf War–deployed, Gulf War–era, and Bosnia-deployed UK veterans who responded to a questionnaire. The authors compared their questionnaire results with the CDC definition of CMI and found that 25.3% of Gulf War veterans, 12.2% of era veterans, and 11.8% of Bosnia-deployed veterans met the criteria. In all three groups of veterans, meeting the CDC case definition was significantly associated with a variety of wartime and environmental exposures (Unwin et al., 1999).

In an evaluation of the CDC definition, Smith et al. (2013) conducted a survey of a sample of 495 veterans drawn from the VA Gulf War Health registry about 10 years after the Gulf War. The study included veterans from all branches of the military and was weighted to be representative of the national population. The investigators asked about 35 symptoms but focused on the 10 main symptoms identified by Fukuda et al. and found that 33.8% met the definition of CMI. They also examined symptoms of postwar onset (excluding those with onset during or before the war), which Fukuda et al. did not require. Requiring onset of symptoms after the war did not change the prevalence (33.4%) substantially. Symptoms found to be most characteristic of CMI cases, in descending order of most commonly reported, are fatigue, memory problems, joint pain, joint stiffness, difficulty in sleeping, moodiness, difficulty with words, depression, muscle pain, and anxiety. Symptoms were endorsed by 55.9% of cases. Finally, the investigators examined agreement between the CDC definition and veterans' beliefs about deployment-related illness: 19.4% met the CMI case definition and believed that they were suffering from CMI, 13.8% of veterans who met the criteria for CMI did not believe that they had CMI, and 14.8% did not meet the CMI criteria but believed that they did have CMI. A similar description of 2,961 UK veterans' beliefs reported that 17.3% believed that they had CMI, and 90% of those fit the CDC CMI criteria (Chalder et al., 2001).

Kansas

The Kansas Persian Gulf Veterans Health Initiative in 1998 sponsored a study of deployment-related symptoms (Steele, 2000). The investigator chose to develop a clinically based descriptive definition using correlated symptoms. To be considered in this study, symptom onset must have been in 1990 or later, and symptoms must have been present in the year before interview. Participants were excluded if they had a diagnosis of or were being treated for cancer, diabetes, heart disease, chronic infectious disease, lupus, multiple sclerosis, stroke, or any serious psychiatric condition.

Gulf War veterans (2,030) who lived in Kansas participated in a telephone interview. Correlated symptoms of veterans who met the study criteria above resulted in five reliable symptom groups: fatigue and sleep problems, pain, neurologic and mood, gastrointestinal, and respiratory symptoms. One symptom, rashes, was not part of the correlation analysis but was frequently reported and correlated with deployment, so it was also included. In all symptom groups, greater symptom burden was associated with deployment. Gulf War veterans reported worse overall health and more symptoms. The proportion of exclusionary conditions was similar in deployed and nondeployed veterans. Notably, Gulf War veterans were more likely than nondeployed veterans to report moderate or multiple symptoms in three or more symptom groups. The author developed a case definition that required

- Symptom onset after 1990.
- The presence of symptoms in the year before the interview.
- No diagnoses or treatment for exclusionary conditions (cancer, diabetes, heart disease, chronic infectious disease, lupus, multiple sclerosis, stroke, or any serious psychiatric condition).
- Symptoms in at least three of six symptom groups: fatigue and sleep problems, pain, neurologic and mood, gastrointestinal, respiratory, and skin symptoms.
- At least one moderately severe symptom or two or more symptoms within a symptom group.

The Kansas case definition resulted in a prevalence of 34.2% in Gulf War veterans and 8.3% in nondeployed veterans (odds ratio [OR] = 4.68, 95% confidence interval [CI] 3.25–6.75); application of the CDC case definition to the same study population definition resulted in a prevalence of 47.2% in Gulf War veterans and 19.8% in nondeployed veterans (OR = 3.26, 95% CI 2.48–4.28). The Kansas definition found CMI more prevalent in women, those with lower income, those with less education, Army veterans, and enlisted personnel.

Portland

Population-based studies supported by the Portland Environmental Hazards Research Program have also proposed a definition of CMI (Bourdette et al., 2001; Spencer et al., 1998). A questionnaire and clinical evaluation assessed symptoms in Gulf War veterans by combat period. The study, conducted in 1998, included 244 cases and 113 controls who were deployed to the Persian Gulf. Participants lived in Oregon or Washington state. Veterans who served in other conflicts, such as Vietnam, were excluded from the study. Cases reported (and confirmed) at least one symptom from among three groups: fatigue, cognitive–psychologic, and musculoskeletal symptoms. Symptoms must have persisted or recurred for a month or longer, must have been present in the 3 months before evaluation, and must have begun during or after deployment to the Persian Gulf. After clinical evaluation, a committee composed of neurologists, rheumatologists, internal-medicine specialists, neuropsychologists, and epidemiologists reviewed each participant and excluded those who had exclusionary disorders and diagnostic explanations for reported symptoms. Exclusionary diagnoses included cancer, epileptic seizures, HIV, schizophrenia, hepatitis, hypothyroidism, alcoholism, effects of shift work, mechanical back pain, myofascial pain, bursitis or tendonitis, patellofemoral syndrome, osteoarthritis, diet intolerance, and diabetes mellitus. Skin and gastrointestinal symptoms were not used to define a case, because they were almost always explained by a diagnosable condition or not present at the time of evaluation. Controls did not report symptoms during or after their military service. Stratification by deployment period revealed no differences in symptoms between precombat, combat, and postcombat periods. However, cases were more likely to score lower on the Armed Forces Qualification Tests, to have served more days in theater on the average, and to have been members of the Army (Spencer et al., 1998). In addition, 48% of cases reported symptoms in two or more symptom groups, and 20% reported symptoms in all three groups.

Another study of the same population performed a factor analysis of the 69 symptoms reported on the questionnaire to determine whether the symptom groups used for the clinical definition described above could approximate the statistical approach of grouping symptoms and to assess potential misclassification of cases and controls on the basis of the clinical definition (Bourdette et al., 2001). The factor analysis supported the clinically described symptom groups, but its identification of cases and controls differed slightly. The factor analysis–derived case definition was congruent with the clinically derived definition, but the selection of cases differed, identifying 10 of 113 controls as cases and 52 of 241 cases as controls.

Department of Veterans Affairs

VA sponsored several studies of the health of Gulf War veterans (Kang et al., 2000, 2002). A followup investigation of the same sample assessed "unexplained multisymptom illness" to describe veterans who had such symptoms as fatigue, muscle or joint pain, headache, memory problems, respiratory problems, and skin problems that persist for more than 6 months and were not adequately explained by established, conventional medical or psychiatric disorders. On the basis of that definition, 36.5% of Gulf War veterans and 11.7% of nondeployed veterans met the case definition. About 75% of Gulf War veterans who had CMI reported that symptom onset occurred during 1991–1995. Those who had CMI reported significantly worse physical and mental functioning than nondeployed veterans. This clinically derived definition of unexplained multisymptom illness had the highest adjusted OR among more than 20 conditions but was not unique to Gulf War veterans (Kang et al., 2009).

TABLE 5.1 Case Definitions of Multisymptom Illness Used in Gulf War Veteran Studies[a]

Definition	Symptoms—must have signs, symptoms, or complaints that fit at least	Duration	Onset	Exclusions	Severity
Haley—clinical (Haley et al., 1997)	5 of 8 signs or symptoms: 1) fatigue 2) arthralgia or low back pain 3) headache 4) intermittent diarrhea without bloody stools 5) neuropsychiatric complaints of forgetfulness, difficulty in concentrating, depression, memory loss, or easy irritability 6) difficulty in sleeping 7) low-grade fever 8) weight loss			Must be denied a physician's diagnosis of other medical and psychiatric illnesses that could cause the symptoms	
Haley—factor analysis (Haley et al., 1997)	Cases are defined mathematically by using factor scores calculated with weights; cases with factor scores >1.5 are identified as having a syndrome (a factor derived with the same factor analysis); cases may have multiple syndromes				
CDC (Fukuda et al., 1998)	1 or more from at least 2 of the following categories: 1) fatigue 2) mood and cognition (symptoms of feeling depressed, difficulty in remembering or concentrating, feeling moody, feeling anxious, trouble in finding words, or difficulty in sleeping) 3) musculoskeletal (symptoms of joint pain, joint stiffness, or muscle pain)	≥6 months			Mild, moderate, or severe by self-report
Kansas (Steele, 2000)	3 of 6 domains: 1) fatigue and sleep problems 2) pain symptoms 3) neurologic, cognitive, and or mood symptoms 4) gastrointestinal symptoms 5) respiratory symptoms 6) skin symptoms	Chronic	Since 1990	Symptom reporting must be in the absence of diagnosed exclusionary conditions; only respondents who have at least 1	Mild, moderate, or severe by self-report

Definition	Symptoms—must have signs, symptoms, or complaints that fit at least	Duration	Onset	Exclusions	Severity
				moderately severe symptom or 2 or more symptoms within a group were considered to have a high level of symptoms in the group	
Portland (Bourdette et al., 2001; Spencer et al., 1998)	Symptoms in 1 of 3 categories: 1) fatigue (unexplained fatigue and at least 4 of the following: fevers and chills; new kinds of headache; unrefreshing sleep; tender glands in the neck, jaw, or groin; changes in memory or difficulty in concentrating; sore throat; painful joints; unexplained weakness in many muscles; persistent muscle aches; prolonged fatigue; and feeling of illness lasting longer than 1 day after mild exercise) 2) cognitive and psychologic symptoms, including memory loss, confusion, inability to concentrate, mood swings, and sleep difficulties 3) musculoskeletal symptoms, including back pain, persistent muscle aches or pains, painful joints, swollen joints, joint stiffness, and pain after exertion	≥1 month within the 3 previous months	During or after deployment to the Persian Gulf War		
VA (Kang et al., 2009)	Might include things like fatigue, muscle or joint pain, headache, memory problems, digestive problems, respiratory problems, skin problems, or any other unexplained symptoms that may sometimes be diagnosed as chronic fatigue syndrome, fibromyalgia, irritable bowel syndrome, or multiple chemical sensitivity	≥6 months		Must not be adequately explained by conventional medical or psychiatric diagnoses	

NOTE: CDC = Centers for Disease Control and Prevention; VA = Department of Veterans Affairs.
[a]Other elements of case definitions (such as laboratory criteria and exposure) not reported.

DISCUSSION OF EXISTING CASE DEFINITIONS

The committee reviewed the literature that identified the symptoms found in Gulf War veterans through questionnaires and surveys, factor analysis, and clinical observation. After a thorough discussion of that literature, the committee concluded that it was not feasible to develop a new evidence-based definition of CMI. The case-definition studies do not all consistently identify period of onset, duration, frequency, severity, exposure, exclusionary criteria, or a uniform set of symptoms. There are no clinically validated tests or measures for diagnosing CMI. Furthermore, the symptoms of CMI are not unique to Gulf War–deployed veterans although they occur in the deployed at a higher frequency and with greater severity than in nondeployed era veterans or those deployed elsewhere. That is evidenced by higher prevalences of a variety of symptoms, as noted in the cohort studies (see Chapter 3) and depicted in the graph in Appendix B. Thus, the committee has concluded that the available evidence is insufficient to develop a new case definition of CMI inasmuch as the data are lacking for key elements of a case definition of a symptom-defined condition, which might include, for example, onset, duration, and measures of severity.

To move the field forward, the committee has developed an approach that is based on its evaluation of the CMI literature and its collective judgment. In its review of CMI symptomatology, factor analyses, and case definitions, the committee noted similarities throughout the body of literature. A common set of symptoms has been identified in *all* the case-definition studies summarized in this chapter (albeit not necessarily using the same terminology) that includes symptoms of fatigue, pain, and neurocognitive dysfunction. Furthermore, the different symptoms in the symptom-based studies—as summarized in Chapter 3, Table 4.2, and Appendix B—were regularly reported with higher frequency in Gulf War veterans than in nondeployed era veterans or veterans deployed elsewhere; they include gastrointestinal, respiratory, and dermatologic symptoms in addition to the fatigue, pain, and neurocognitive symptoms already identified. The committee recognized that two *existing* definitions—the CDC definition and the Kansas definition (see Table 5.1)—capture the array of symptoms most commonly identified. The CDC definition requires one or more symptoms in at least two of the categories of fatigue, pain, and mood and cognition to identify a case. The Kansas definition requires at least three of six symptoms in the domains of fatigue–sleep, pain, neurological–cognitive–mood, gastrointestinal, respiratory, and skin to identify a case. Thus, both definitions capture the array of symptoms highlighted by the evidence. The CDC case definition, which has been widely used by researchers, identifies 29–60% of US Gulf War–deployed veterans as CMI cases, depending on the population studied, whereas the Kansas definition identifies 34% of the population studied (Kansas Gulf War veterans) (see Table 5.2).

The two definitions have important differences. The CDC definition has the greatest concordance with all the other definitions (see Table 5.1) but is less restrictive than the Kansas definition. The CDC definition requires fewer symptoms, does not include any exclusionary criteria, and might identify a case without physical symptoms. The Kansas definition will define fewer veterans as cases. The committee also noted particular strengths of each definition, including the CDC definition's inclusion of severity indicators and the Kansas definition's exclusionary criteria.

In the committee's judgment, neither definition has been sufficiently validated. Given the absence of validators, the committee recommends, with some reticence, the use of two current case definitions. The CDC and Kansas definitions are the best reflection of the symptom complexes demonstrated by the Gulf War veterans. The committee recognizes that the definitions were developed in different study populations and that they differ in sensitivity and specificity. However, in the committee's judgment, those two definitions will provide the VA with a framework that will further research and treatment.

TABLE 5.2 Reported Prevalence of CMI

Study	CMI Rate (%) GWVs	NDVs	Definition	Period of Data Collection	Population
Fukuda et al. (1998)	45%	15%	CDC	1995	Air Force units
Wolfe et al. (2002)	60%		CDC	1997–1998	Ft. Devens cohort
Unwin et al. (1999)	62%	36%	CDC	1998	UK veterans
Chalder et al. (2001)	59%		CDC	1998	UK veterans
Kelsall et al. (2009)	26%	16%	CDC	2000–2002	Australian veterans
Smith et al. (2013)	34%		CDC	~2001	US national sample of GWVs
Blanchard et al. (2006)	29%	16%	CDC	2001	US national sample of GWVs
Steele (2000)	34%	8%	Kansas	1998	Veterans in Kansas
Kang et al. (2009)	37%	12%	VA	2005	US national sample of GWVs
Haley et al. (1997)	25%		Haley FA	1994–1995	A Seabee reserve battalion
Haley et al. (1997)	34%		Haley clinical	1994–1995	A Seabee reserve battalion
Haley et al. (2001)	29%		Haley FA	1997–1998	US Army veterans living in north Texas
Iannacchione et al. (2011)	14%	4%	Haley FA	2007–2009	US national sample of GWVs

NOTE: CDC = Centers for Disease Control and Prevention; CMI = chronic multisymptom illness; FA = factor analysis; GWV = Gulf War veteran; NDV = nondeployed veteran; VA = Department of Veterans Affairs.

In conclusion, the committee saw merits in both the CDC and Kansas definitions, but the weight of the evidence does not support use of one rather than the other for all purposes. Given the differences, the committee notes the importance of choosing a definition that is based on specific needs. For example, the CDC definition may not be suitable for research that requires a more narrowly defined study population whereas the Kansas definition may identify too few cases and compromise statistical power. Another consideration in choosing a definition is the ability to adapt a definition that is suitable for use in clinical settings.

CONCLUSIONS

After reviewing the literature on Gulf War veterans' symptoms the committee came to several conclusions:

- The 1990-1991 Gulf War presented a unique set of circumstances and experiences to the Gulf War veterans.
- They symptoms complex as described by numerous researchers resembles previous war syndromes.
- The evidence to date does not indicate that there is a unique Gulf War syndrome as many of the symptoms experienced by Gulf War veterans are also experienced by the non-deployed and deployed elsewhere.
- Gulf War veterans report more symptoms and more severe symptoms than the non-deployed or deployed elsewhere populations.
- The symptom reporting is similar in Gulf War veterans from the US, Canada, UK, Denmark, and Australia.
- There is no universally accepted case definition and none of the current definitions meet the general criteria of case definitions (e.g., onset, duration, severity, exclusionary criteria).
- The available evidence is insufficient to develop a new case definition.

RECOMMENDATIONS

Evidence is lacking in the studies reviewed to characterize most elements of a case definition (for example, onset, duration, severity, and laboratory findings) with certainty. Without that information, the committee could not develop a new definition for CMI. Furthermore, because that information is lacking, few of the studies that proposed definitions were able to describe many of the elements of a case definition. Although all the studies describe clinical features (symptoms), many of the other criteria are not discussed. Therefore, the committee cannot recommend one specific case definition over another. But it does recommend the consideration of two case definitions on the basis of their concordance with the evidence and their ability to identify specific symptoms commonly reported by Gulf War veterans.

There is a set of symptoms (fatigue, pain, neurocognitive) that are reported in all the studies that have been reviewed. The CDC definition captures those three symptoms; the Kansas definition also captures them, but it also includes the symptoms reported most frequently by Gulf War veterans (see Appendix B). Other case-definition studies report additional symptoms that are not seen with the same frequency or in all studies. Thus, the committee identified the CDC definition (Fukuda et al., 1998) and the Kansas definition (Steele, 2000) as the two that capture the array of symptoms most frequently reported by veterans as evidenced by the studies reviewed (see Chapter 3 and Appendix B).

The committee recommends that the Department of Veterans Affairs consider the use of the Centers for Disease Control and Prevention and Kansas definitions because they capture the most commonly reported symptoms.

Neither definition addresses all the key features of a case definition, such as, symptom onset, duration, severity, frequency of symptoms, and exclusionary criteria. Identifying those features will contribute to a more accurate case definition. Those features were not regularly reported in the studies considered. It is important to acknowledge that the two definitions, although they cover the most common symptoms, do not reflect the complete array of symptoms reported by Gulf War veterans. Although a standard set of criteria regarding time (a defined period of onset), place, exposures, and clinical and laboratory findings would have been useful; given the lag in time between first reports of illness and epidemiologic study, lack of exposure monitoring, and the absence of validated laboratory tests, it is no longer possible to define many of the typical elements associated with a case definition. However, review of existing data sets might prove useful in detailing some of the needed information.

The committee recommends that the Department of Veterans Affairs, to the extent possible, systematically assess existing data to identify additional features of chronic multisymptom illness, such as onset, duration, severity, frequency of symptoms, and exclusionary criteria to produce a more robust case definition.

Finally, VA asked the committee to evaluate the terminology used in referring to CMI in 1990–1991 Gulf War veterans and to recommend appropriate terminology. Multiple terms have been used over the past 2 decades. Initially, *Gulf War syndrome* was used, but *syndrome* indicates a new group of signs and symptoms not previously seen in medicine (IOM, 2000; King's College London, 2010). The Gulf War veterans report more symptoms and with greater frequency and severity than nondeployed veterans or veterans who were deployed elsewhere, but the types and patterns of symptoms are the same in all groups, and this suggests that no unique syndrome is associated with Gulf War deployment.

Although *chronic multisymptom illness* is descriptive of the heterogeneity of the symptoms, it is not specific to the population and its unique experience. Thus, to capture the population of interest and the symptoms, a preferred term is *Gulf War illness*. Illnesses are sometimes named after the geographic area or the group in which they were first identified without meaning to convey a sole etiology (for example, the 1918 influenza pandemic referred to as the Spanish flu, the 1968 and 1969 influenza outbreaks referred to as the Hong Kong flu, and pneumonia in legionnaires referred to as Legionnaire's disease). The committee's recommendation reflects both the geographic area and the unique experiences of this group of veterans. *Gulf War illness* has been used by many researchers to identify the array of symptoms expressed by Gulf War veterans. Its consistent use in the literature might reduce confusion.

The committee recommends that the Department of Veterans Affairs use the term *Gulf War illness* rather than *chronic multisymptom illness*.

CONSIDERATIONS FOR FUTURE RESEARCH

It has been more than 2 decades since the Gulf War, and research has left important questions about the veterans' health unanswered. The inherent limitations of the research and the lack of data regarding exposures are apparent. Additional new research focused on the definition of CMI is likely to be of little, if any, benefit to the veterans. The veteran population is aging, with an associated increase in comorbidities; with the continued passage of time, recall bias is likely to increase. To inform a case definition, a prospective study design with well-defined cohorts that could be systematically characterized with respect to subjective symptoms would have been needed. Symptoms would be characterized according to standardized scales and measures that would also include severity and time of onset. In addition, baseline and prospective collection of biospecimens, accurate exposure monitoring, and pre-deployment and post-deployment health assessments would add to the knowledge base and possibly enable linkages to be made, for example, regarding exposure. Repeated followup of the cohort would enable the systematic characterization of the natural history of the illness and the documentation of changes in symptoms. However, given the passage of more than 20 years, such a study is no longer possible. More fruitful research efforts might focus on identifying subsets of Gulf War veterans who have distinct symptoms and physiologic characteristics with a view to developing effective treatments to improve function and quality of life.

The committee's review revealed a number of limitations in the data that could be reduced in research on future deployments, such as the following:

- Systematic and standardized assessments of frequency, severity, onset, and duration of symptoms in the course of data collection would strengthen the analytic processes.
- Early in the evolution of postdeployment studies, when unexpected magnitudes of veteran complaints occur, more attention to in-depth assessment of subsets of veterans would be valuable.
- A systematic effort to collect and preserve exposure data (such as data on vaccinations, drugs, and environmental exposures) should increase the ability to analyze and interpret reported symptoms. Successful development of a case definition will depend on accurate information about related exposures.

REFERENCES

Blanchard, M. S., S. A. Eisen, R. Alpern, J. Karlinsky, R. Toomey, D. J. Reda, F. M. Murphy, L. W. Jackson, and H. K. Kang. 2006. Chronic multisymptom illness complex in Gulf War I veterans 10 years later. *American Journal of Epidemiology* 163(1):66-75.

Bourdette, D. N., L. A. McCauley, A. Barkhuizen, W. Johnston, M. Wynn, S. K. Joos, D. Storzbach, T. Shuell, and D. Sticker. 2001. Symptom factor analysis, clinical findings, and functional status in a population-based case control study of Gulf War unexplained illness. *Journal of Occupational and Environmental Medicine* 43(12):1026-1040.

Chalder, T., M. Hotopf, C. Unwin, L. Hull, K. Ismail, A. David, and S. Wessely. 2001. Prevalence of Gulf War veterans who believe they have Gulf War syndrome: Questionnaire study. *British Medical Journal* 323(7311):473-476.

Forbes, A. B., D. P. McKenzie, A. J. Mackinnon, H. L. Kelsall, A. C. McFarlane, J. F. Ikin, D. C. Glass, and M. R. Sim. 2004. The health of Australian veterans of the 1991 Gulf War: Factor analysis of self-reported symptoms. *Journal of Occupational and Environmental Medicine* 61(12):1014-1020.

Fukuda, K., R. Nisenbaum, G. Stewart, W. W. Thompson, L. Robin, R. M. Washko, D. L. Noah, D. H. Barrett, B. Randall, B. L. Herwaldt, A. C. Mawle, and W. C. Reeves. 1998. Chronic multisymptom illness affecting Air Force veterans of the Gulf War. *Journal of the American Medical Association* 280(11):981-988.

Haley, R. W., T. L. Kurt, and J. Hom. 1997. Is there a Gulf War syndrome? Searching for syndromes by factor analysis of symptoms. *Journal of the American Medical Association* 277(3):215-222. [Erratum appears in *Journal of the American Medical Association* 1997; 278(5):388.]

Haley, R. W., G. D. Luk, and F. Petty. 2001. Use of structural equation modeling to test the construct validity of a case definition of Gulf War syndrome: Invariance over developmental and validation samples, service branches and publicity. *Psychiatry Research* 102(2):175-200.

Hallman, W. K., H. M. Kipen, M. Diefenbach, K. Boyd, H. Kang, H. Leventhal, and D. Wartenberg. 2003. Symptom patterns among Gulf War registry veterans. *American Journal of Public Health* 93(4):624-630.

Iannacchione, V. G., J. A. Dever, C. M. Bann, K. A. Considine, D. Creel, C. P. Carson, H. Best, and R. W. Haley. 2011. Validation of a research case definition of Gulf War illness in the 1991 US military population. *Neuroepidemiology* 37(2):129-140.

IOM (Institute of Medicine). 2000. *Gulf War and Health, Volume 1: Depleted Uranium, Pyrodostigmine Bromide, Sarin, Vaccines*. Washington, DC: National Academy Press.

Kang, H. K., B. Li, C. M. Mahan, S. A. Eisen, and C. C. Engel. 2009. Health of US veterans of 1991 Gulf War: A follow-up survey in 10 years. *Journal of Occupational and Environmental Medicine* 51(4):401-410.

Kang, H. K., C. M. Mahan, L. Y. Lee, C. A. Magee, and F. M. Murphy. 2000. Illnesses among United States veterans of the Gulf War: A population-based survey of 30,000 veterans. *Journal of Occupational and Environmental Medicine* 42(5):491-501.

Kang, H. K., C. M. Mahan, K. Y. Lee, F. M. Murphy, S. J. Simmens, H. A. Young, and P. H. Levine. 2002. Evidence for a deployment-related Gulf War syndrome by factor analysis. *Archives of Environmental Health* 57(1):61-68.

Kelsall, H. L., D. P. McKenzie, M. R. Sim, K. Leder, A. B. Forbes, and T. Dwyer. 2009. Physical, psychological, and functional comorbidities of multisymptom illness in Australian male veterans of the 1991 Gulf War. *American Journal of Epidemiology* 170(8):1048-1056.

King's College London. 2010. *King's Centre for Military Health Research: A Fifteen Year Report. What Has Been Achieved by Fifteen Years of Research into the Health of the UK Armed Forces?* University of London.

Ozakinci, G., W. K. Hallman, and H. M. Kipen. 2006. Persistence of symptoms in veterans of the first Gulf War: 5-year follow-up. *Environmental Health Perspectives* 114(10):1553-1557.

Rayhan, R. U., M. K. Ravindran, and J. N. Baraniuk. 2013. Migraine in Gulf War illness and chronic fatigue syndrome: Prevalence, potential mechanisms, and evaluation. *Frontiers in Physiology* 4:181.

Smith, B. N., J. M. Wang, D. Vogt, K. Vickers, D. W. King, and L. A. King. 2013. Gulf War illness: Symptomatology among veterans 10 years after deployment. *Journal of Occupational and Environmental Medicine* 55(1):104-110.

Spencer, P. S., L. A. McCauley, S. K. Joos, M. R. Lasarev, T. Schuell, D. Bourdette, A. Barkhuizen, W. Johnston, D. Storzbach, M. Wynn, and R. Grewenow. 1998. U.S. Gulf War veterans: Service periods in theater, differential exposures, and persistent unexplained illness. Portland Environmental Hazards Research Centre. *Toxicology Letters* 102-103:515-521.

Steele, L. 2000. Prevalence and patterns of Gulf War illness in Kansas veterans: Association of symptoms with characteristics of person, place, and time of military service. *American Journal of Epidemiology* 152(10):992-1002.

Unwin, C., N. Blatchley, W. Coker, S. Ferry, and et al. 1999. Health of UK servicemen who served in Persian Gulf War. *Lancet* 353(9148):169-178.

Wolfe, J., S. P. Proctor, D. J. Erickson, and H. Hu. 2002. Risk factors for multisymptom illness in us Army veterans of the Gulf War. *Journal of Occupational and Environmental Medicine* 44(3):271-281.

A

ADDITIONAL INFORMATION ABOUT FACTOR ANALYSIS AND CLUSTER ANALYSIS

This appendix describes factor analysis (FA) and cluster analysis in greater depth than was presented in Chapter 4. Many studies have conducted statistical analysis, predominantly factor analyses but also cluster analysis, to determine whether veterans' symptoms might constitute a new syndrome. By comparing patterns of symptoms and severity between groups of veterans (typically deployed vs nondeployed), some researchers have sought to detect differences that would indicate a deployment-related change. Although many of the statistical analyses have been conducted to inform development of a case definition, they alone do not create a definition. The following pages explain latent variables, FA and related methods, cluster analysis, and structural equation modeling.

LATENT VARIABLES

Latent variables are variables that are not measured directly but are measured indirectly by using observed variables. A latent variable and its observed indicator variables make up a measurement model. There are four basic types of latent variable measurement models: FA, latent class analysis (LCA), latent trait analysis, and latent profile analysis. They can be organized on the basis of whether the *observed variables* are categorical or continuous and whether the *latent variable* is categorical or continuous. LCA models are composed of a categorical latent variable and observed variable whereas FA models are composed of continuous latent and observed variables (Bartholomew and Knott, 1999). There are other types of latent variable models, but for simplicity they are not discussed here. In medicine, syndromes (sets of symptoms that occur together more often than expected by chance alone) can be modeled as latent variables. In those cases, the observed indicator variables are the reported symptoms, and the latent variable is the hypothesized, but unknown, underlying disorder. The two types of latent variable models used most commonly in medicine are FA and LCA.

FACTOR ANALYSIS

FA is a statistical technique developed for data reduction and for developing scales and identifying latent relations among variables. More specifically, an FA evaluates the intercorrelation among variables within a dataset. FA can be conceptualized as a set of linear regressions solved simultaneously, in which each observed variable is a dependent variable in a linear regression, each latent factor is an independent variable, and the loadings are regression coefficients. It is assumed that the relationships between the factors and the observed variables are linear, and that there are no interactions among the observed variables.

FA cannot be used for "identifying" or "discovering" factors. Similarly, it would be inappropriate (and misleading) to refer to factors as "emerging" from a factor analysis. Such terminology inaccurately implies that there is a "true" set of factors underlying the data and that this factor set need only be unearthed. In fact, factor-analytic results are seldom unequivocal and are influenced by a series of analytic decisions. It should be noted that the editor's comment in a 2009 paper on FA of symptoms in Gulf War veterans (Kang et al., 2002, 68) points out that "factor analysis is not completely objective; for example, there are no definite rules for selecting the appropriate number of factors . . . or rules for selecting from among the many possible methods of rotation. It is an empirical method."

Another misunderstanding of FA is the confusion of its goal with the goal of cluster analysis (Stewart, 1981). The goal of factor analysis is to suggest a structure that explains the relationships among variables in a dataset, not to identify item clusters or posit groups of people. Because the hypothesized structure typically includes substantially fewer factors than items, FA is considered a data-reduction technique. Instead of explaining the data on the basis of responses to each individual item or symptom, a data structure is posited that is more parsimonious.

Variables for Factor-Analytic Studies

The data for FA studies may be people's responses to a set of items from a questionnaire or list of symptoms. They may include dichotomous items (such as yes–no questions) or items with more than two response options (such as never–sometimes–always). In the case of chronic multisymptom illness (CMI), responses to both kinds of items have been factor-analyzed. For example, Hom et al. (1997) asked participants to indicate the presence or absence of 50 physical and psychologic symptoms, and Forbes et al. (2004) asked respondents to rate the intensity of 63 symptoms as "mild," "moderate," or "severe."

When using an FA software program, the analyst typically enters individual responses to each item (for example, one row for every respondent and as many columns as there are items). The software compares each item with other items one at a time and calculates the correlation of responses on every pair of items. Rather than entering individual response data, the analyst may enter the intercorrelation matrix itself. Table A.1 shows a hypothetical intercorrelation matrix for a dataset that included responses to six items. Typically, one would not conduct an FA on the basis of such a small number of variables, but it is presented for discussion purposes. In viewing the matrix in Table A.1, one will note that it is *symmetrical*: the numbers above the diagonal are mirror images of those below it. In addition, the numbers in the diagonal are all 1.000, representing the correlation between an item and itself. That is pointed out because, as will be explained later, in some FA approaches, the 1.000 is replaced with a different number. In the FA studies on CMI, many more items were used. Knoke et al. (2000), for example, conducted FA of responses to 98 items. The intercorrelation matrix for such an analysis would have contained 98 rows and 98 columns.

FA is not a single method but a family of analytic strategies that includes, for example, exploratory factor analysis (EFA) and confirmatory factor analysis (CFA). EFA is used to identify the underlying relationships among a large number of variables when there is no a priori hypothesis. CFA is a hypothesis-driven approach.

TABLE A.1 Hypothetical Intercorrelation Matrix for a Six-Item Dataset

	Item 1	Item 2	Item 3	Item 4	Item 5	Item 6
Item 1	1.000	0.362	0.313	0.208	0.299	0.445
Item 2	0.362	1.000	0.671	0.208	0.550	0.432
Item 3	0.313	0.671	1.000	0.346	0.587	0.706
Item 4	0.208	0.208	0.346	1.000	0.681	0.606
Item 5	0.299	0.550	0.587	0.681	1.000	0.347
Item 6	0.445	0.432	0.706	0.606	0.347	1.000

The Factor-Analysis Family of Methods

As explained below, an investigator conducting an FA faces a number of decision points and must decide among several options at each. They include decisions about factor extraction, rotation, the number of factors to retain, and whether to drop items. With the availability of user-friendly software and its generous use of default values, it is possible to complete an FA and not be aware of the need to make such decisions. But default decisions are decisions, nonetheless, and it is important to understand their ramifications.

Factor Extraction

One distinction among FA methods is the statistical approach used in "factor extraction." Two of the available choices are reviewed, common FA and principal component analysis (PCA). To date, all published FA studies of CMI have used one of those two methods.

In FA, the variance in individual responses to items is assumed to be one of three types: common variance (shared variance), the portion of variance in a variable (for example, survey item) that is shared with one or more other variables; unique variance, the portion of variance that is specific to a single variable; and error variance, the variance not explained in the FA model. Both common FA and PCA are methods for analyzing the variance within a dataset. In FA, however, only the shared or "common" variance is targeted; in a PCA, all the variance in scores is analyzed. That difference in strategy reflects the differing purposes of FA and PCA. FA attempts to identify the structure of the common variance within a dataset. It is the method often (not always) chosen for scale development when the interest is in identifying the scalable, latent domains that best explain the variance in scores (Worthington and Whittaker, 2006). PCA, in contrast, targets the total variance in scores and attempts to represent all the variance, not just the common variance, in scores. There is no consensus as to which approach is "better"; in fact, FA and PCA often yield similar results (Velicer and Jackson, 1990). Complicating the choice is that there are variations even within methods. FA methods include, for example, image, principle-axis, and maximum-likelihood factoring (Tabachnick and Fidell, 2001).

The differences among the submethods of FA and PCA are beyond the scope of this report, but it is important to document the choices when publishing FA results. That applies to all the decision points in an FA.

In the course of an FA study, investigators may conduct multiple FA (for example, comparing a three-factor and a two-factor solution) and compare the resulting hypothesized structures. The choice of the optimal number of factors to extract is based on a number of considerations. Historically, "scree" plots, the amount of variance explained by the factors, and eigenvalues were used. More recently, parallel analysis has been recognized as a superior method (Hayton et al., 2004). It operates by generating a user-specified number of simulated datasets that have the same number of variables as the observed dataset; each variable has the same mean and standard deviation as its analogous variable in the observed dataset. The difference is that in the simulated datasets the variables are uncorrelated. PCA is conducted on each of the simulated datasets, and a component (factor) is retained only if the eigenvalue for the component exceeds the mean of the eigenvalues for the component from the simulated datasets.

After the number of factors to extract is chosen, typically the solution is rotated to produce solutions that are more easily interpreted (for example, when items load more strongly on one factor and weakly or not at all on all other factors). A number of different rotations are possible, and they affect the interpretation, but not the fit, of the model. The rotation methods produce factors that are either orthogonal (factors are forced to be uncorrelated with each other) or oblique (factors are allowed to be correlated with each other). The decision as to whether to allow the factors to be correlated should be based on substantive theory: Are the latent variables correlated with each other in the conceptual model? Many of the published FA of CMI used orthogonal rotations (such as varimax), and this forced an assumption of unrelatedness of the factors.

So far, the models that have been described have been types of EFA; in these models, each variable is allowed to load on each latent factor. To simplify the model, researchers often follow their EFA models with CFA models in which each item is allowed to load on only one factor. Fitting such a model is mathematically equivalent to imposing an assumption that each observed variable has only one nonzero factor loading.

Confirmation of Model Structure

Because the summary variables resulting from FA are latent (unobserved) and the product of a number of (often subjective) decisions, it is important that an FA be replicated. When sample size permits, that can be done by splitting the dataset in two before any analysis and retaining half for confirmation. It is also helpful to replicate a factor solution in an independent sample. In those cases, the goal is to demonstrate "measurement invariance"; this means that the observed variables in the model can be used to measure the latent constructs of interest in the same way in different samples.

There are a number of levels of measurement invariance to indicate whether factor loadings are the same. The first is configural invariance. If, in two samples analyzed independently, the same number of factors is chosen as optimal, and each observed variable loads on the same factors in both samples, then configural invariance has been achieved. Second, One would then determine whether the loadings of each item on each factor are the same in the two samples. That is done by fitting two models: in the first, the loadings are allowed to be estimated freely; in the second, the loadings are forced to be identical in the two samples. The two models will be nested, and their fit can be compared via a likelihood ratio test or chi-squared difference test to determine whether the constrained model fits significantly worse. If so, measurement invariance cannot be claimed.

Occasionally, researchers will fit a CFA model derived from a previous sample in a new sample and assess its fit by using common metrics, such as the Tucker-Lewis Index and comparative fit index (Hu and Bentler, 1999). It is important to note that demonstrating acceptable fit in the new sample is not sufficient to demonstrate measurement invariance. One must first demonstrate configural invariance by replicating the EFA.

In some cases, further levels of measurement invariance are explored, including ones that require that not only the loadings but the residual variance be identical among samples. Such a level of measurement invariance is seldom achieved, however, and it is not typically considered necessary.

LATENT CLASS ANALYSIS

In LCA measurement models, a number of latent groups (classes) are proposed. People are assumed to be a member of one and only one class, in such a way that the probabilities of membership in all of the classes sum to 1. For example, if there are two latent classes, and the probability of being in the first class is 0.75, the probability of being in the second class must be 0.25. Those probabilities are referred to as latent class probabilities. Each of the latent classes is characterized by different probabilities of having each of the symptoms related to the condition of interest. For example, if CMI is a homogenous condition with less symptom variability and a LCA model were fitted to data from every service member deployed during the Gulf War, one would expect a two-class model. The first class would be relatively asymptomatic, with low or nearly zero probabilities of each of the symptoms associated with CMI. The second class would have higher rates of each of those symptoms. These probabilities are referred to as conditional probabilities because they vary as a function of class membership. Because CMI is not homogenous and symptoms are highly variable, one would expect to use a model with three or more classes. For example, if there were both neurologic and respiratory variants of CMI, one would expect a three-class model with one class of relatively asymptomatic people, a second class with high conditional probabilities of the neurologic symptoms but low probabilities of other symptoms, and a third class with high conditional probabilities of the respiratory symptoms but low probabilities of other symptoms.

Like FA, LCA entails assumptions of independent people and local independence. In the present context, the assumption of independent people implies that there is no clustering of people and that one person's pattern of symptoms is not related to another's. Gulf War veterans were clustered within units and may have shared exposures. Furthermore, people in a given unit may have discussed their symptoms with their fellows. For example, a soldier might be more likely to report a symptom that he would otherwise have dismissed if he knew that a number of other soldiers in his unit also experienced that symptom. For that reason, the assumption of independent people may be problematic. Hierarchic modeling techniques, which account for such clustering, have been developed for both FA and LCA.

In the context of the Gulf War symptom literature, the assumption of local independence implies that when a person's latent class membership is accounted for, the probability of having a given symptom is not affected by whatever other symptoms the person has. For example, in the sample as a whole, two respiratory symptoms, coughing and shortness of breath, will certainly correlate; that is, people who cough are more likely to have shortness of breath than the sample as a whole. If there were a respiratory class, local independence would imply that *among people who are members of the respiratory class*, a person's probability of having shortness of breath would be the same regardless of whether he or she experienced coughing.

FA requires a decision on the part of the analyst regarding the number of latent factors to extract. Analogously, LCA requires a decision regarding the number of latent classes to fit. Typically, models with successively larger numbers of classes are fitted, and the model that has the fewest classes while still accounting for associations among the observed indicator variables (symptoms) is chosen (Nylund et al., 2007). As in FA, the decision has a subjective element, and the model and its results can vary dramatically on the basis of the decision.

Unlike FA, which groups symptoms along a number of axes, LCA groups people into latent classes. After a model is fitted, the estimated latent class probabilities, conditional probabilities, and each person's pattern of symptoms can be used to calculate each person's probability of being in each class. It is important to note that class membership is latent, so it is possible to say only that on the basis of this person's pattern of symptoms, he or she is *most likely* to be a member of class x.

FA has both exploratory and confirmatory variants; LCA has no such analogue. Confirmation of the latent class model would entail replicating both the number of classes and the conditional probability estimates for each class. A formal test of measurement invariance would entail fitting the latent class model in two separate samples. If the same number of latent classes appeared optimal in both samples, one would then compare two models: a model in which the conditional probabilities for each symptom for each class were allowed to be different between the two samples and a model in which they were forced to be the same. The first model will always fit better because it is specifically tailored for each sample. The question is, How much better? That can be tested mathematically by using a likelihood ratio test because the two models are nested (the second, constrained model can be represented as a special case of the first model). If the test is statistically significant, one rejects the constrained model and concludes that the two samples differ in their underlying latent class structure. In lay terms, one can think of a model fitting data in the way that a set of clothes fits a person. One way to determine whether you have the same body shape and size as another person would be to ask how you look in your own clothes and compare it with how you look when you try on that person's clothes. If you look *significantly* worse, you will reject the hypothesis that you have the same body shape.

LCA has not been used to model CMI. That may be because LCA is newer; computer programs capable of estimating such models were not available until the late 1980s and have become widely available only in the past 10–15 years. Some of the commonly used software programs—including SPSS, SAS, and STATA—still do not have this capability as part of their base packages, unlike MPLUS and R. FA, in contrast, has been available for some time in all these packages. Another barrier to the use of LCA is the relatively large samples required (Muthén and Muthén, 2002). That is due partly to the nature of the data on which the analyses operate. The input for FA is a triangular matrix of correlations between indicator variables. In the case of 50 indicator variables, that would mean 1,225 separate values in the triangular matrix. In contrast, the input for LCA is the numbers of people who have each possible pattern of symptoms. An analysis that includes 50 dichotomous symptoms results in more than a quadrillion (2^{50}) possible symptom patterns. For that reason, LCA typically use fewer than 15 indicator variables.

LCA is potentially useful in the study of CMI because its goal is to group people, and it is preferable to post hoc processes of grouping people on the basis of their unvalidated factor score cutoffs. However, researchers using LCA to model CMI would have to make potentially difficult decisions about which symptoms to include in the model.

CLUSTER ANALYSIS

There are several methods of cluster analysis; however, because all cluster analysis studies included in this report use k-means methodology the discussion below is limited k-means cluster analysis. K-means cluster analysis is a method of grouping people that has been used to model CMI data. Cluster analysis is not a latent-variable method; it does not assume that an underlying latent variable accounts for any associations between observed variables. Instead, cluster analysis is a type of computational learning method that aims to find clusters that are not known in advance. The "K" in the name denotes the number of clusters to be estimated, and this quantity is supplied by the analyst. Given a fixed number of clusters, the algorithm finds the points in p-dimensional space for each of the *K* clusters that minimizes the sum of the distances from each point to the nearest centroid (the center of each cluster). Figure A.1 shows an example in which two clusters are estimated by using people's values for each of three observed symptoms. In contrast with LCA, in which class membership is latent, in cluster analysis people are placed into clusters as part of the estimation process, and cluster membership can be treated as an observed variable. Although the process is computationally intensive, it is capable of handling larger numbers of symptoms than LCA. Until recently, a major drawback of cluster analysis was that the choice of number of clusters to estimate could be quite subjective. However, the recently developed gap statistic has been shown to perform well in choosing the number of clusters (Tibshirani et al., 2001). In Addition, variable selection in cluster analysis can be determined in a variety of ways (Steinly, 2006). A remaining drawback is that methods of replication and validation of cluster structures are still an open field of methodologic research. Furthermore, because cluster analysis is not a latent-variable method, it is not possible to incorporate cluster membership within a larger structural equation framework, as one could with either FA or LCA.

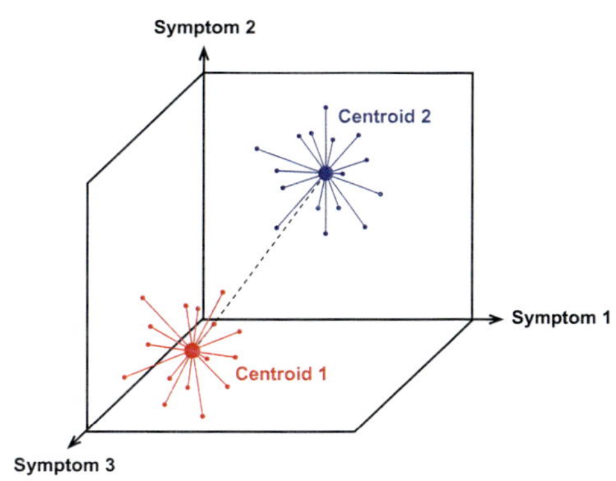

FIGURE A.1 Example of two clusters based on three symptoms.

STRUCTURAL-EQUATION MODELING

Once a latent-variable measurement model is estimated, the next step is to attempt to validate the measurement. In this context, validity implies that the measurement of the variable is equal to the true value of the variable on the average. For example, to validate your bathroom scale as a measurement of your weight, you would compare it with your true weight as measured with a gold standard. That process is relatively straightforward for two reasons: first, there is a gold standard for weight, and second, the definition of weight is well understood and agreed-on.

Validating measures of latent variables is considerably less straightforward because there are generally no gold standards, and the nature of a latent variable itself is often in question. In such cases, the best option is to assess whether the measurement of the latent variable is consistent with current theory regarding the latent variable and its relationships with other variables (Cronbach and Meehl, 1955).

In the context of developing a case definition of CMI, the case definition itself can be thought of as an instrument for determining whether a person has CMI. If there were a gold standard for CMI, it would be possible to assess the sensitivity (the probability that a person who has CMI meets the case definition), specificity (the probability that a person who does not have CMI does not meet the case definition), positive predictive value (the probability that a person who meets the case definition has CMI), and negative predictive value (the probability that a person who does not meet the case definition does not have CMI). All four of those values could be used to judge the performance of the case definition as a measure of CMI. Today, there is no gold standard, and such calculations are not possible. The next best option is to develop a theory-based network of observed variables that should be related to CMI. The most obvious variable is patient history of deployment and history of exposures; additional variables might include patient characteristics and results of diagnostic tests. It is assumed that if the case definition is a valid measure of CMI, "caseness" will be associated with those variables, and that such associations can be taken as evidence in support of the validity of the case definition.

Structural-equation models can be used to model associations with latent variables. In those models, associations are estimated jointly with the measurement model (such as the factor analysis or latent class analysis). Because they are modeled jointly, it is possible for the associated variables to influence the formation of the measurement model. That can be helpful in that it means that all available data are used to model the latent variable. However, if the goal is confirmation of the measurement model, it may be preferable to "fix" the measurement model and then to assess the relationships between the measurement model and the validating variable. In such cases, it is inappropriate to treat the latent variable as though it had been directly observed; special procedures are necessary to ensure an unbiased estimate between the latent variable and the validating variable (Nyland et al., 2007). Failure to correct for such biases can result in a missed association; it may appear that a validating variable is not associated with a latent variable even though it actually is associated.

LOOKING FORWARD

FA, LCA, and cluster analysis may be useful methods for making sense of the large number of symptoms potentially associated with CMI. However, the findings from these models must be validated against other observed variables. The process may involve multiple iterations in which observed validating variables are used to refine a measurement model and make possible more accurate assessment of the associations between the measurement model and the observed variables; that in turn further refines the measurement model. Such an iterative process could lead to identification of biomarkers of CMI, which in turn would inform research on mechanisms and treatment. The process could also be used to identify or rule out putative causes. Given that there are a variety of potential causes, which may have acted in concert, it will be important to explore relationships among risk factors and to incorporate the findings into the models.

Latent-variables models, like any other models, are only as good as the data that are used to fit them. The choice of variables to include in a measurement model is critical, and omission of key symptoms will result in models that do not capture the most salient features of CMI. Data on exposures, risk factors, and symptoms have been collected almost solely on the basis of self-reports. Verification of exposures after the fact may not be possible, but it is possible to assess the test–retest reliability of exposure self-reports. For example, did people who reported taking pyridistigmine bromide tablets 5 years after deployment also report having taken them 10 years after deployment? If reports have not been consistent, care should be taken in interpreting findings based on such data.

REFERENCES

Bartholomew, D. J., and M. Knott. 1999. *Latent Variable Models and Factor Analysis*. Vol. 7. New York: Arnold.

Cronbach, L. J., and P. E. Meehl. 1955. Construct validity in psychological tests. *Psychological Bulletin* 52(4):281-302.

Forbes, A. B., D. P. McKenzie, A. J. Mackinnon, H. L. Kelsall, A. C. McFarlane, J. F. Ikin, D. C. Glass, and M. R. Sim. 2004. The health of Australian veterans of the 1991 Gulf War: Factor analysis of self-reported symptoms. *Journal of Occupational and Environmental Medicine* 61(12):1014-1020.

Hayton, J., D. G. Allen, and V. Scarpello. 2004. Factor retention decisions in exploratory factor analysis: A tutorial on parallel analysis. *Organizational Research Methods* 7(2):191-205.

Hom, J., R. W. Haley, and T. L. Kurt. 1997. Neuropsychological correlates of Gulf War syndrome. *Archives of Clinical Neuropsychology* 12(6):531-544.

Hu, L., and P. M. Bentler. 1999. Cutoff criteria for fit indicies in co variance structure analysis: Conventional criteria versus new alternatives. *Structural Equation Modeling* 6(1):1-55.

Kang, H. K., C. M. Mahan, K. Y. Lee, F. M. Murphy, S. J. Simmens, H. A. Young, and P. H. Levine. 2002. Evidence for a deployment-related Gulf War syndrome by factor analysis. *Archives of Environmental Health* 57(1):61-68.

Knoke, J. D., T. C. Smith, G. C. Gray, K. S. Kaiser, and A. W. Hawksworth. 2000. Factor analysis of self-reported symptoms: Does it identify a Gulf War syndrome? *American Journal of Epidemiology* 152(4):379-388.

Muthén, L. K., and B. Muthén. 2002. How to use a monte carlo study to decide on sample size and determine power. *Structural Equation Modeling* 9(4):599-620.

Nyland, K. L., T. Asparouhov, and B. O. Muthén. 2007. Deciding on the number of classes in latent class analysis and growth mixture modeling: A monte carlo simulation study. *Structural Equation Modeling* 14(4):535-569.

Steinley, D. 2006. K-means clustering: A half-century synthesis. *British Journal of Mathematical and Statistical Psychology* 59(1):1-34.

Stewart, D. W. 1981. The application and misapplication of factor analysis in marketing research. *Journal of Marketing Research* 18:51-62.

Tabachnick, B. G., and L. S. Fidell. 2001. *Using Multivariate Statistics, Fourth Edition*. Boston, MA: Allyn and Bacon.

Tibshirani, R., G. Walther, and T. Hastie. 2001. Estimating the number of clusters in a data set via the gap statistic. *Journal of the Royal Statistical Society: Series B* 63, part 2:411-423.

Velicer, W. F., and D. N. Jackson. 1990. Component analysis versus common factor analysis: Some issues in selecting appropriate procedures. *Multivariate Behavioral Research* 25(1):1-28.

Worthington, R. L., and T. A. Whittaker. 2006. Scale development research: A content analysis and recommendations for best practices. *The Counseling Psychologist* 34:806-838.

B

PERCENTAGES OF VETERANS REPORTING SYMPTOMS IN STUDIES OF GULF WAR VETERANS AND MILITARY PERSONNEL

The following graph depicts the percentages of veterans who endorse symptoms as reported in studies cited in Chapter 3. The minimum, median, and maximum are indicated for each category of symptoms. Data are further characterized by whether the reports came from deployed Gulf War personnel and veterans (GWVs), nondeployed Gulf War–era personnel and veterans (NGVs), and Gulf War–era personnel and veterans deployed to other regions (Else). The percentages do not represent prevalence inasmuch as the results of all study types (including military-based and registry studies) cited are not representative of the population. Groups of symptoms are listed along the vertical axis, and the horizontal axis displays the percentage of veterans endorsing the symptoms.

Figure B.1 is followed by additional detail, including the number of times (N) that a symptom was reported in GWVs, and a description of the symptoms in each category as reported by studies. It should be noted that some studies report multiple symptoms in a group; for example, both vomiting and diarrhea are included in gastrointestinal (GI) symptoms and are reported separately by some studies and together in others. Also, the number of studies that reported symptoms in each group varies; for example, many studies reported on cognitive symptoms, fewer on chemical sensitivity. The numbers of symptoms reported by individual studies also vary. Each bar represents a different number of studies, and each bar represents a collection of symptoms.

For NGVs and Else, fewer studies reported percentages for a given symptom. For example, nine studies reported symptoms of allergies in GWVs, eight in NGVs, and one in Else.

Figure B.1 does not differentiate by type of study, number of participants, year, onset, duration, severity, exposure, or other aspects.

Studies that did not report percentages or reported on a study population previously described are not included. And symptoms or symptom groups with five or fewer percentages reported for GWVs are not included in Figure B.1; instead, those symptoms or symptom groups are listed in Table B.1.

FIGURE B.1 Range and median of percentages of veterans reporting symptoms in studies of Gulf War veterans and military personnel.

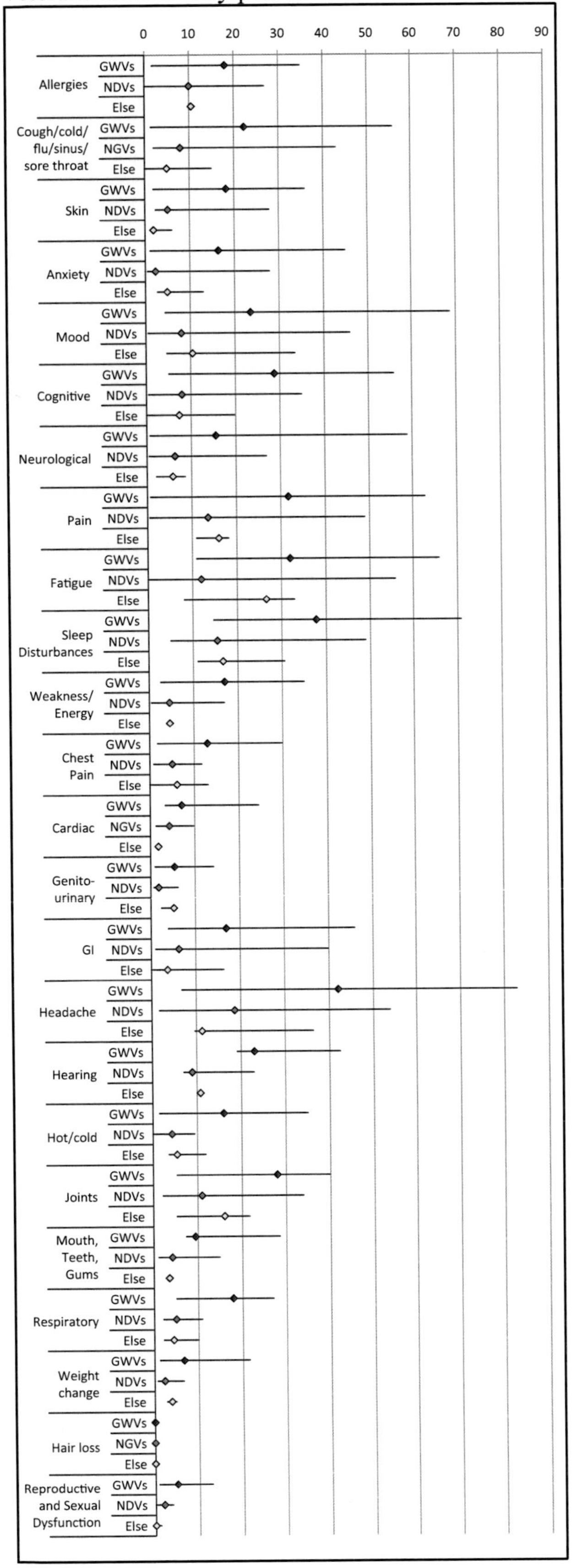

NOTE: Else = veteran deployed elsewhere; GI = gastrointestinal; GWV = Gulf War veteran; NGV = nondeployed veteran.

SOURCES: Doebbeling et al., 2000; Fukuda et al., 1998; Gray et al., 1999, 2002; Iowa Persian Gulf Study Group, 1997; Ishøy et al., 1999; Joseph et al., 1997; Kang et al., 2000; Kelsall et al., 2004; Kroenke et al., 1998; Nisenbaum et al., 2004; Proctor et al., 1998; Roy et al., 1998; Salamon et al., 2006; Simmons et al., 2004; Steele et al., 2012; Stretch et al., 1995; Unwin et al., 1999; Wolfe et al., 1998.

The terminology used by study authors to describe symptoms is listed below for each group of symptoms with the number of percentages in GWVs reported (N). There were several symptoms that fit easily into the symptom groups or symptom groups with five or fewer percentages reported in GWVs (see Table B.1).

Allergies (N = 9): hay fever or allergies (>6 months); hay fever or allergies; allergic edemas of face, eyes, or lips; allergic eye symptoms; itchy painful eyes; allergies (other than skin); allergies.

Cough/cold/flu/sinus/sore throat (N = 36): bothered by cough; cough; cough (>6 months); persistent cough; persistent cough when don't have cold; continual cough; common cold or flu; flu; head colds; congested/mucous or phlegm; sinus troubles; sinus congestion (>6 months); sinus congestion; runny nose; sore throat; symptoms of bronchitis.

Skin (N = 20): rash; rashes; rash or sores (>6 months); skin rashes; skin rash; rash or skin ulcer; skin irritation; rash or skin irritation; dryness or scaling of skin; skin rashes, eczema, skin allergies; skin allergies; eczema; sensations of itching on skin; other forms of skin problems; moderate or multiple skin symptoms.

Anxiety (N = 20): nervous or tense; feeling anxious (>6 months); frequent periods of anxiety or nervousness; anxious; chronic anxiety; chronic worry/anxiety; panic or anxiety; feeling of nervousness, irritability, or agitation; feeling jumpy/easily startled; symptoms of anxiety disorder; symptoms of posttraumatic stress disorder (PTSD); PTSD and associated symptoms; anxiety/stress/sleep disturbance; taking medication to sleep or calm down; nightmares/flashbacks; nightmares; distressing dreams.

Mood (N = 40): depression; depressed; depressed mood; depression or sadness; feeling depressed (>6 months); feeling down or depressed; frequent periods feeling depressed; symptoms of major depression; symptoms of minor depression; any symptoms of depression; symptoms of chronic dysphoria; crying easily; feeling distant or cut off; avoiding doing things or situations; feeling life is pointless, meaningless; loss of interest; loss of interest in TV, movies, news, friends; mood swings, aggression, irritability; irritability; unusual irritability; unusual anger; irritability or outbursts of anger; feeling irritable/angry outbursts; moody, irritable (>6 months); frequent rage.

Cognitive (N = 43): loss of concentration; difficulty concentrating; difficulty remembering or concentrating (>6 months); concentration or memory difficulties; memory difficulties; memory loss; memory loss/lack of concentration; memory problems; problems with memory; short-term memory problems; problems remembering recent information; difficulties leaning new information; problems with forgetfulness; forgetfulness; difficulty finding the right word; difficulty to find words; difficulty with speech; disturbances of speech, trouble finding and pronouncing words correctly; trouble finding words (>6 months); trouble finding words when speaking; confusion; episodes of disorientation (>6 months); feeling disoriented; symptoms of cognitive dysfunction.

Neurological (N = 42): dizziness or trouble maintaining balance (>6 months); dizziness; dizziness or feeling lightheaded; feeling dizzy, lightheaded, or faint; balance disturbances or fits of dizziness; blurred or double vision; blurred vision; blurred vision not improved by the use of glasses; double vision; eyes very sensitive to light; increased sensitivity to light; increased sensitivity to noise; numbness; numbness in arms or legs; numbness or tingling; numbness or tingling (>6 months); numbness or tingling in extremities; numbness or tingling in fingers or toes; numbness or tingling in hands or feet; numbness or tingling in parts of body; numbness/tingling/dizziness; tingling in fingers and arms; tingling in legs and arms; tingling or shivering of arms, legs, or other parts of the body; shaking; tremors or shaking; tremors/shaking; muscle twitches or trembling; moderate or multiple neurologic symptoms; other neurological or neuromuscular not otherwise specified (NOS).

Pain (N = 45): body pain/hurt all over; general aches and pains; general muscle aches and pains; muscle aches/cramps; muscle pain; muscle pain (>6 months); muscle tension, aches, soreness, or stiffness; muscular pain/weakness; pain in muscles; unusual muscle pain; joint pain; joint pain (>6 months); joint pains; pain in joints; roving joint pain; pain without swelling or redness in several joints; aching joints/bones; pain or ache in more than one joint; back ache, low back pain, neckaches or stiffness; back problems; moderate or multiple pain symptoms; symptoms of fibromyalgia.

Fatigue (N = 33): fatigue; all fatigue; fatigue (>6 months); unusual fatigue; unusual feeling of fatigue during the day; fatigue lasting 24 hours after exertion (>6 months); fatigue lasting 24 hours; problems with fatigue lasting more than 24 hours after having made a physical effort; abnormal feeling of fatigue (not caused by physical activity); extreme fatigue every day, or almost every day; moderate or multiple fatigue symptoms; excessive sleepiness; sleepiness; sleepy all the time; needed more rest; feeling unrefreshed after sleep; feeling unusually sleepy/drowsy; feeling unwell after exercise/exertion; awakening with a feeling of fatigue and exhaustion after a hole night's sleep; problems with feeling tired; symptoms of chronic fatigue.

Sleep disturbances (N = 19): sleep disturbance; sleeping difficulties; difficulty sleeping (>6 months); difficulty sleeping; trouble sleeping; inability to fall asleep; problems falling asleep; problems falling or staying asleep; trouble falling or staying asleep; problems sleeping all night; not feeling rested after sleep; unrefreshing sleep.

Weakness/energy (N = 8): feeling weak in parts of your body; generalized muscle weakness; general muscle weakness; loss of strength; suddenly diminished muscular power; lacking energy; overly tired/lack of energy.

Chest pain (N = 11): chest pain (>6 months); chest pain; chest pain/tightness; tightness in chest.

Cardiac (N = 12): rapid heartbeat; rapid heart rate; rapid heart rate (not exercising); racing heart; irregular heartbeats or "hear flutters"; irregular heartbeat; blood pressure; heart problems.

Genitourinary (N = 10): passing urine more often; frequent urination; frequent or painful urination; frequent, painful urination; pain on passing urine; urinary infections; kidney disease/symptoms; genital system and bladder problems.

GI (gastrointestinal) (N = 54): diarrhea; diarrhea (>6 months); frequent diarrhea; recurrent diarrhea; loose or aquaeous stools; diarrhea or constipation; constipation; alternating loose and hard stools; flatulence or burping; gas, bloating, cramps, abdominal pain (>6 months); rumbling in the stomach more than a couple of times a week; nausea; nauseous; nausea or vomiting (>6 months); nausea, vomiting; vomiting, nausea, or upset stomach; nausea, upset stomach; stomach upset; upset stomach; stomach ache; stomach cramp; abdominal pain; abdominal pain or cramping; stomach cramps or excessive gas; stomach pain/ulcer; dyspepsia or esophageal disease; heartburn; gastralgia; irritated bowel syndrome; moderate or multiple GI symptoms; digestive symptoms.

Headache (N = 21): any headaches; headache; headache (>6 months); headaches; recurrent headaches; repeated fits of headache; severe headache.

Hearing (N = 7): loss of hearing or ringing in ears; ringing in ears; tinnitus; audition disorders; hearing loss.

Hot/cold (N = 17): chills; chills/fever; feeling feverish; fever; fever (>6 months); fever or chills; hot or cold spells, fever, sweats, chills; low tolerance for heat or cold; night sweats; night sweats that soak bed sheets (>6 months); night sweats that soak the bed sheets; night sweats/excessive; sweating/fevers; sweating.

Joints (N = 11): joint stiffness; joint stiffness (>6 months); joint swelling; swelling in joint; joint swelling/redness.

Mouth, teeth, gums (N = 8): problems with mouth gums or teeth; mouth/gum problems; problems with teeth or gums; bleeding gums; teeth loss; mouth sores.

Respiratory (N = 25): difficulty breathing or catching breath; difficulty breathing or shortness of breath; unable to breathe deeply enough; shortness of breath; shortness of breath (>6 months); shortness of breath (not exercising); feeling short of breath at rest; dyspnea; dyspnea or cough; wheezing; wheezing (>6 months); wheezing in chest; rapid breathing; faster breathing than normal; moderate or multiple respiratory symptoms; symptoms of asthma.

Weight change (N = 13): weight gain/loss; sudden weight gain; unintended weight gain ≥10 lbs; appetite loss/weight loss; sudden weight loss; weight loss; unintended weight loss ≥10 lbs; unintended weight loss ≥10 lbs (>6 months).

Hair loss (N = 7): hair loss; unusual hair loss; sudden hair loss; any hair loss or hair disease.

Reproductive and sexual dysfunction (N = 13): painful intercourse; pain during intercourse; problems during sexual intercourse; decreased interest in sex (>6 months); sexual dysfunction/lack of sex drive; impotence; burning semen; burning in sex organs; veteran or partner feels a burning sensation after sex; menstrual difficulties.

TABLE B.1 Symptoms Not Included in Figure B.1 (≤5 Reported Percentages per Symptom or Symptom Group)

Symptom	Study	% GWVs Reporting Symptom	% NGVs Reporting Symptom	% Deployed Elsewhere Reporting Symptom
Alcohol: symptoms of alcohol abuse; intolerance to alcohol	Nisenbaum et al., 2004; Schwartz et al., 1997	19.4–11.9	4–16.8	5.0
Appetite: appetite loss; loss or decrease in appetite	Gray et al., 2002; Nisenbaum et al., 2004	9.4–13.3	3.0–5.2	3.4–8.5
Chemical sensitivity: chemical sensitivity; chemical sensitivity (>6 months); multiple chemical sensitivity; sensitive to chemicals; symptomatic response to chemicals, odors	Fukuda et al., 1998; Gray et al., 2002; Kang et al., 2000; Salamon et al., 2006; Steele et al., 2000	4.3–17.0	0.7–8.0	0.7
Chronic/frequent infection	Simmons et al., 2004	5.8	1.6	
Deterioration of general health	Simmons et al., 2004	3.7	2.9	
Difficulty in swallowing: problems swallowing; trouble with swallowing; difficulty swallowing	Kang et al., 2000; Salamon et al., 2006; Stretch et al., 1995	12.1–16.2	5.0–7.2	
Eyes, ears, nose: eyes trouble; eyes, ears, nose trouble; nasal sores (>6 months)	Salamon et al., 2006; Stretch et al., 1995	17.0–26.0	5.5–5.6	
Hoarseness	Stretch et al., 1995	9.7–12.0	4.1–3.7	
Injuries and healing: retarded wound healing; bruise easily; tendency to bruise or bleed easily; slowness of healing; slow healing	Ishoy et al., 1999; Kang et al., 2000; Salamon et al., 2006	3.5–13.0	1.7–7.0	
Lump in throat	Nisenbaum et al., 2004	8.0	3.0	3.80
Milk intolerance (>6 months)	Fukuda et al., 1998	7.0	4.0	
Nuisances after vaccination	Ishoy et al., 1999	2.8	0.0	
Other: other; other symptoms; other symptoms not otherwise specified	Joseph et al., 1997; Roy et al., 1998; Simmons et al., 2004; Stretch et al., 1995	5.1–21.4	1.9–6.5	
Reporting ≥1 symptom	Simmons et al., 2004	60.7	36.7	
Single episodes of acute infections	Simmons et al., 2004	2.7	2.0	
Skeletal and other muscular symptoms	Simmons et al., 2004	15.1	13.2	
Suicidal thoughts	Gray et al., 2002	6.4	2.7	2.6
Sweaty clammy or damp hands	Ishoy et al., 1999; Wolfe et al., 1998	7.0–7.9	3.9	
Swelling of feet	Kang et al., 2000	11.0	6.0	
Swollen glands: sore or swollen glands in neck; swollen glands; swollen lymph nodes (>6 months)	Fukuda et al., 1998; Kang et al., 2000; Salamon et al., 2006; Steele et al., 2000	8.0–17.7	2.0–8.0	
Tendency to bruise or bleed easily	Salamon et al., 2006	3.5		

REFERENCES

Doebbeling, B. N., W. R. Clarke, D. Watson, J. C. Torner, R. F. Woolson, M. D. Voelker, D. H. Barrett, and D. A. Schwartz. 2000. Is there a Persian Gulf War syndrome? Evidence from a large population-based survey of veterans and nondeployed controls. *American Journal of Medicine* 108(9):695-704.

Fukuda, K., R. Nisenbaum, G. Stewart, W. W. Thompson, L. Robin, R. M. Washko, D. L. Noah, D. H. Barrett, B. Randall, B. L. Herwaldt, A. C. Mawle, and W. C. Reeves. 1998. Chronic multisymptom illness affecting Air Force veterans of the Gulf War. *Journal of the American Medical Association* 280(11):981-988.

Gray, G. C., K. S. Kaiser, A. W. Hawksworth, F. W. Hall, and E. Barrett-Connor. 1999. Increased postwar symptoms and psychological morbidity among U.S. Navy Gulf War veterans. *American Journal of Tropical Medicine and Hygiene* 60(5):758-766.

Gray, G. C., R. J. Reed, K. S. Kaiser, T. C. Smith, and V. M. Gastanaga. 2002. Self-reported symptoms and medical conditions among 11,868 Gulf War-era veterans. *American Journal of Epidemiology* 155(11):1033-1044.

Iowa Persian Gulf Study Group. 1997. Self-reported illness and health status among Gulf War veterans: A population-based study. *Journal of the American Medical Association* 277(3):238-245.

Ishøy, T., P. Suadicani, B. Guldager, M. Appleyard, H. O. Hein, and F. Gyntelberg. 1999. State of health after deployment in the Persian Gulf. The Danish Gulf War study. *Danish Medical Bulletin* 46(5):416-419.

Joseph, S. C., R. R. Blanck, G. Gackstetter, R. Glaser, K. C. Hyams, S. Kinty, C. Magruder, J. Mazzuchi, F. L. O'Donnell, M. D. Parkinson, R. E. Patterson, and D. H. Trump. 1997. A comprehensive clinical evaluation of 20,000 Persian Gulf War veterans. *Military Medicine* 162(3):149-155.

Kang, H. K., C. M. Mahan, L. Y. Lee, C. A. Magee, and F. M. Murphy. 2000. Illnesses among United States veterans of the Gulf War: A population-based survey of 30,000 veterans. *Journal of Occupational and Environmental Medicine* 42(5):491-501.

Kelsall, H. L., M. R. Sim, A. B. Forbes, D. C. Glass, D. P. McKenzie, J. F. Ikin, M. J. Abramson, L. Blizzard, and P. Ittak. 2004. Symptoms and medical conditions in Australian veterans of the 1991 Gulf War: Relation to immunisations and other Gulf War exposures. *Journal of Occupational and Environmental Medicine* 61(12):1006-1013.

Kroenke, K., P. Koslowe, and M. Roy. 1998. Symptoms in 18,495 Persian Gulf War veterans: Latency of onset and lack of association with self-reported exposures. *Journal of Occupational and Environmental Medicine* 40(6):520-528.

Nisenbaum, R., K. Ismail, S. Wessely, C. Unwin, L. Hull, and W. C. Reeves. 2004. Dichotomous factor analysis of symptoms reported by UK and US veterans of the 1991 Gulf War. *Population Health Metrics* 2.

Proctor, S. P., T. Heeren, R. F. White, J. Wolfe, M. S. Borgos, J. D. Davis, L. Pepper, R. Clapp, P. B. Sutker, J. J. Vasterling, and D. Ozonoff. 1998. Health status of Persian Gulf War veterans: Self-reported symptoms, environmental exposures and the effect of stress. *International Journal of Epidemiology* 27(6):1000-1010.

Roy, M. J., P. A. Koslowe, K. Kroenke, and C. Magruder. 1998. Signs, symptoms, and ill-defined conditions in Persian Gulf War veterans: Findings from the comprehensive clinical evaluation program. *Psychosomatic Medicine* 60(6):663-668.

Salamon, R., C. Verret, M. A. Jutand, M. Begassat, F. Laoudj, F. Conso, and P. Brochard. 2006. Health consequences of the first Persian Gulf War on French troops. *International Journal of Epidemiology* 35(2):479-487.

Simmons, R., N. Maconochie, and P. Doyle. 2004. Self-reported ill health in male UK Gulf War veterans: A retrospective cohort study. *BMC Public Health* 4:1-10.

Steele, L., A. Sastre, M. M. Gerkovich, and M. R. Cook. 2012. Complex factors in the etiology of Gulf War illness: Wartime exposures and risk factors in veteran subgroups. *Environmental Health Perspectives* 120(1):112-118.

Stretch, R. H., P. D. Bliese, D. H. Marlowe, K. M. Wright, K. H. Knudson, and C. H. Hoover. 1995. Physical health symptomatology of Gulf War-era service personnel from the states of Pennsylvania and Hawaii. *Military Medicine* 160(3):131-136.

Unwin, C., N. Blatchley, W. Coker, S. Ferry, M. Hotopf, L. Hull, K. Ismail, I. Palmer, A. David, and S. Wessely. 1999. Health of UK servicemen who served in Persian Gulf War. *Lancet* 353(9148):169-178.

Wolfe, J., S. P. Proctor, J. D. Davis, M. S. Borgos, and M. J. Friedman. 1998. Health symptoms reported by Persian Gulf War veterans two years after return. *American Journal of Industrial Medicine* 33(2):104-113.